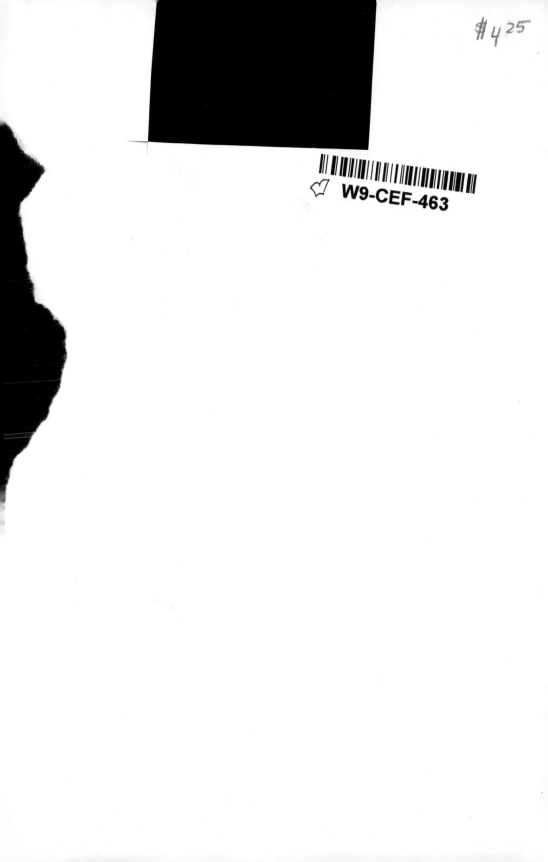

MIRACLE BOY GROWS UP

MIRACLE BOY GROWS UP
HOW THE DISABILITY RIGHTS REVOLUTION SAVED MY SANITY

BEN MATTLIN

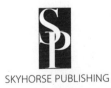

SKYHORSE PUBLISHING

Skyhorse Publishing books may be purchased in bulk at special discounts for sales promotion, corporate gifts, fund-raising, or educational purposes. Special editions can also be created to specifications. For details, contact the Special Sales Department, Skyhorse Publishing, 307 West 36th Street, 11th Floor, New York, NY 10018 or info@skyhorsepublishing.com.

Skyhorse® and Skyhorse Publishing® are registered trademarks of Skyhorse Publishing, Inc.®, a Delaware corporation.

Visit our website at www.skyhorsepublishing.com.

10 9 8 7 6 5 4 3 2 1

Library of Congress Cataloging-in-Publication Data

Mattlin, Ben, 1962-
 Miracle boy grows up : how the disability rights revolution saved my sanity / by Ben Mattlin.
   p. cm.
 ISBN 978-1-61608-731-9 (hardcover : alk. paper)
 1. Mattlin, Ben, 1962- 2. Spinal muscular atrophy--Patients--United States--Biography. 3. People with disabilities--United States--Biography. 4. Authors with disabilities--United States--Biography. 5. People with disabilities--Civil rights--United States. 6. Social movements--United States. I. Title.
 RC935.A8M38 2012
 617.4'82044092--dc23
 [B]
                                2012017734

Printed in the United States of America

FOR MY FAMILY OF ORIGIN
AND MY FAMILY NOW—

I am truly fortunate.

"No matter what we have come through, or how many perils we have safely passed, or how imperfect and jagged—in some places perhaps irreparably—our life has been, we cannot in our heart of hearts imagine how it could have been different."

—Randolph S. Bourne, *Youth And Life*
(Chapter VI: "The Adventure of Life")

CONTENTS

Introduction ix

CHAPTER 1: Two Roads Diverged in Apartment 2B 1

CHAPTER 2: Disability as a Social Condition 9

CHAPTER 3: Divorce, Bar Mitzvahs, and Preadolescence—
Wasn't My Life Hard Enough? 25

CHAPTER 4: My Unfortunate, Life-Changing Incarceration 43

CHAPTER 5: The End of Childhood. 60

CHAPTER 6: *Maman Est Morte* 76

CHAPTER 7: What I Gained and Lost in College 92

CHAPTER 8: If No One Notices a Disability,
Does It Really Exist? 108

CHAPTER 9: Becoming More Disabled 128

CHAPTER 10: Nesting. 146

CHAPTER 11: The Bubble Bursts. 164

CHAPTER 12: The Ghanaian Connection. 178

Introduction

My new attendant's first day starts with basic training: how to wash me ("first the soap . . . "), dress me ("slide one foot into the jeans leg, then the other . . . "), and lift me from bed into my wheelchair ("put one hand under my knees and the other behind my back and lift me like a groom carries a bride over the threshold . . . ").

A UCLA student from Ghana, Africa, Jerry had answered my classified ad in the *Daily Bruin*, the university newspaper, for a morning attendant. The *Bruin* is my latest favorite attendant source. Its circulation spans the local community, and its classifieds supply staff to many nearby restaurants and doctors' offices. Something about being just another area employer appeals to me.

Since my last attendant quit several months ago—the group home for retarded adults, his other job, demanded more of him—I've been eager to find a replacement but didn't want to be too hasty either. I know the right guy can improve my mood, my productivity, my family's quality of life. I don't know why attendants have this power over me. Doubtless it has to do with their being such a constant presence, to the extent that they function as my arms and legs. Perhaps it's also because they always used to be older than I am; I saw them as surrogate big brothers or even fathers. Now that I'm nearly forty-four,

I should be in the daddy role. I should have more natural authority. Maybe it'll go better from now on.

My first impression of Jerry was the proper résumé he'd e-mailed, which is unheard of in this line of work. He'd then arrived on time for his interview, neatly shutting the door behind him, which I always watch for as a sign of not just tidiness but a sense of personal responsibility. He'd proffered a hand, and I as usual said something like "can't reach you, but I'm pleased to meet you." He'd calmly proceeded to lower himself onto our sofa, pushing up his glasses and pulling up his loose-fitting, low-slung jeans.

I always try to imagine how it will be seeing this person early in the morning, when I'm not awake enough to want to see anybody. Jerry looked scruffy—long dreadlocky hair and a ragged beard of sorts, like many young men these days.

"How are you today?" he'd asked, presenting a typed list of references, which is impressive in itself. "And what would you like to know about me?"

No obvious accent, which reassured me there's a fair chance of good verbal communication. For me that's essential, since I can't point or otherwise demonstrate physically what I need.

Jerry has just transferred to UCLA. He's twenty-five and on a student visa. He works evenings with troubled high school kids. He likes helping people— his goal is to get a good education and go back to his country to help institute social reforms and keep the peace—but has never worked with disabled people or in any kind of medical setting.

That's the way I like it. I don't want to be called "the patient." Those with any kind of background in the field tend to think they know what's best for me. They don't. Not all of us who ride in wheelchairs are the same.

"Your ad said 'will train,' and I like that," he'd said next, smiling. "When you say you need me to shave you, for example, you can explain how?"

"Yes," I'd answered, thinking *I've found my man.*

I told him I'd check his references and be back in touch shortly. It may sound like a dodge, but I always check references. In the past, I've uncovered all kinds of unforgivable dirt. His turned out to be stellar. A few days later I offered him the position—two hours every weekday. That's all I could afford at the moment.

After a successful first day, while tying my shoes, Jerry asks a question that's dangerously close to my tolerance boundary: "How do you stay so positive?"

It's just baby steps from calling me inspirational. Which I'm used to, of course, but still. "I don't, and I'm not," I answer. "Just doing what I gotta do."

The next day he again comments on how much he enjoys my "positivity" and wonders what keeps me going.

"Necessity," I say sarcastically.

"There's so much anger out there," he goes on, undeterred. "I work with high school kids who have trouble functioning because they're so filled with anger. You don't get angry?"

"Sure. Wait till you know me longer."

Gradually, it sinks through my self-righteous emotional shield, burnished by the disability-rights movement to rebuff all but the most specific forms of praise. There's something different about what he's saying. My earnest young employee is commenting not about something over which I've no control—the fact that I've lived my whole life with a severe neuromuscular condition—but about my attitude, an attitude I've adopted and nurtured, a doggedly honed personality trait, a survival strategy, perhaps. He might've asked the same question if I didn't have a disability!

How have you survived this sometimes rough world?

I could've asked him the same question. An immigrant from a poor country, working his way through school, dedicated to helping others. What drives *him*? (Another odd realization: This time the attendant is inspiring *me*!)

Usually the "you're so inspirational" business is followed by something like, "You should write a book about your life. It would be *so* inspirational for so *many* people! Then you could go on *Oprah*!" Which turns me off. Nothing against Oprah, but let survivors of abuse, cancer, or war coax tears from readers' eyes. Not me.

Yet Jerry doesn't resort to the book-and-Oprah spiel. Not exactly. What he does do, that morning and for many others that follow, is get me talking. And that's when I realize something. I do have a lot to say. And I do have a personal history that's not the same as everybody else's. It's a story of luck and persistence, by turns ordinary and extraordinary. And, upon further reflection, I come to see how closely my story tracks a surge of unprecedented advances in medicine, technology, and civil rights that people with disabilities have enjoyed and harnessed. Indeed, the synchronicity between that movement and my own is surely more than coincidental.

Maybe it's my age. There comes a point when you get too old to care what other people think. Perhaps I've at last reached a level of maturity from where I can look back at my varied experiences with unself-conscious honesty and feel nothing but humbled and grateful.

And if it happens to inspire people, that's *their* problem!

CHAPTER ONE

TWO ROADS DIVERGED IN APARTMENT 2B

1962–1966

"I am not my body; my body is nothing without me."
—Tom Stoppard, *Rock 'n' Roll*

In 1962, some 4 million babies were born in the US—nearly 700 of them with an undiagnosed neurological disorder that will gradually weaken their muscles until, in most cases, breathing becomes too difficult, pumping blood becomes impossible, and they die.

I am one of the 700.

Though hereditary and therefore genetically present at birth, spinal muscular atrophy—as it's now known—can remain invisible until late-childhood or even adulthood. Mine shows up before I'm six months old. Half of those who manifest symptoms in infancy die before they reach the age of two. Their hearts and lungs become too weak to go on.

I am one of the lucky ones.

By the time I'm six months old, my mother has already noticed I'm not progressing as my older brother Alec did. I can't sit up by myself. When placed in a sitting position, I fall over. After I bang my head on the parquet countless times, my parents stop sitting me on the floor. They sit me on the sofa instead, surrounded by pillows. They sit me in a high chair, where I can be strapped in. Later, they put a small football helmet on me, especially when I try to balance on my rocking horse or tricycle, or when Alec and I roughhouse. It's too heavy, however, and makes staying upright even harder.

My parents know something is wrong, but they don't know what.

They ask the pediatrician, who refers them to a specialist. The specialist recommends another specialist. And so on. The months become years, during which I am paraded before countless physicians, therapists, researchers, and even a few crackpots. No faith healers (thank God!); my parents are not praying people. Still, I wouldn't be surprised if they offered up a few silent ones during the long waits in hushed waiting rooms and perhaps in the dead of night.

Even in the twenty-first century, when SMA is well known among neurologists, there's no slowing or stopping it. It's now considered the most common cause of genetically based neonatal death. It's estimated that one in every 6,000 Americans is born with a form of it, and one in 40 carries the gene that causes it without ever manifesting symptoms. In comparison, approximately one in every 300 Americans is HIV-positive, and one in every 206 has some form of cancer, according to the Centers for Disease Control and Prevention. SMA is more common than, say, ovarian cancer, which strikes one in every 8,065 American women (including my mother and maternal grandmother).

Not until the 1990s do researchers finally zero in on the exact genetic mechanism behind SMA. Most cases stem from a faulty gene on the fifth chromosome, which results in a deficiency of what's called SMN1, a necessary protein. This deficiency, in turn, depletes motor-nerve cells in the spinal cord. But certain instances of infantile SMA have a different culprit—a mutation of a gene called UBE1, which happens to be on the X chromosome. This mutation impedes the disposal of a bad protein, allowing it to flourish. I don't know which version causes my SMA. In either case, these markers make SMA scientifically identifiable and *may* someday lead to effective treatments.

But in the '60s, when I'm a child, SMA is undiagnosable and, perhaps consequently, considered extremely rare by those who have heard of it at all.

So I'm at first diagnosed with many other conditions. Spina bifida. Brain damage. Mental retardation. That last one invariably coaxes a chuckle from my dad later, in the retelling: "Those *doctors* were retarded!" In my cerebral family, God forbid you should make fun of the *physically* handicapped—and don't dare say "cripple"—but the mentally retarded are fair game.

One thing all the doctors and sundry experts agree upon, however, in the early '60s: I'm a "floppy baby." I have what's called "floppy-baby syndrome." It's still a recognized pathology in medical dictionaries. I lack muscle tone.

A more scientific-sounding word for lacking muscle tone is "amyotonia," and that's what becomes my first official diagnosis. I learn to say "amyotonia" before I can add two and two. For me, it's a way of understanding my body—a plausible answer for the strangers who point at me and ask, "What's wrong with him?"

Or more often, "What's wrong with *her*?" The blond curls and long eyelashes I sport in those days apparently emasculate me. Never "What's wrong with *you*?" I'm not considered competent to answer such a question myself until I'm at least seven.

Nothing is wrong with me! I just have amyotonia, I think to myself. My typical spoken answer, once I'm old enough and courageous enough to speak up: "I can't walk. I was born this way." It seems simpler and sufficient.

I can't walk or stand on my own. When I'm four, my doctors prescribe a battery of physical therapy; as part of it I'm fitted with heavy, metal leg braces. The braces lock me into a statue-straight posture. I'm then placed in a large wooden box, which supports my standing frame. I do this for an hour, three times a week, to aid circulation and overall well-being, or something. It's the closest a modern American child can come to foot binding—yet it's still recommended for many kids in wheelchairs! Luckily for me, the standing therapy is rescinded in a matter of months, when it's determined to have no value. Nevertheless, other physical therapy exercises continue.

In nearly every other aspect I'm a healthy and happy kid. Yet every time I catch a cold I'm at high risk for pneumonia. I can't cough with sufficient force to clear mucus from my lungs. Regardless, from an early age I refuse to think of myself as fragile. Sure, I'm floppy and do bump my head a lot, but I always bounce back. I'm tough, resilient. I'm a survivor. The labors of my disability strengthen my character.

Other remedies are offered from time to time by physicians, therapists, and outspoken streetcorner healers: Massive doses of vitamin E. Transplants of sheep blood. And, of course, acceptance of Jesus Christ as my savior. For the most part my parents resolutely favor modern medical science, but in those days even the legit experts come up abashedly empty-handed. For one thing, my symptoms keep defying expectations.

Specifically, I don't die.

***

"Today my little brother fell out of his wheelchair and dropped his fire engine."

This is what Alec writes in his first-grade composition book one spring weekend when I'm three. He writes it after Dad takes me to the Lamston's under our apartment, on York Avenue at 79th Street in New York City. It's one of my first outings in my shiny new green-upholstered wheelchair. Up till then much of my life experience is from the perspective of Mom's slim hip, Dad's long arms, a baby stroller or the sofa, wedged with pillows. But soon I'll be starting nursery school—at Riverside Church, the only regular nursery school in the city that will take a physically handicapped kid in 1966—so I have to get a proper wheelchair.

I like Lamston's. I've been there before. Our housekeeper / baby-nurse Inez has taken Alec and me a few times. Inez is strict. She's what I understand is called an Egro. She and other Egro baby nurses and maids meet at the Lamston's lunch counter to eat and smoke and gossip.

Today Dad says I can buy a toy at Lamston's if I'll be quiet and behave. It's not hard to choose. I want a Matchbox car. When Dad is done shopping, I remind him of his promise and he pushes me to the toy aisle. But the Matchboxes are on a high shelf. Too high for me to see well from my wheelchair. Dad undoes my seat belt and lifts me up for a better look. He's strong and tall, and with him I feel safe and have no restrictions.

I pick a small fire engine. I don't have any in my collection, and I want one because fire engines can go anywhere. They have no boundaries.

Dad buys it for me, and I clutch the little hook-and-ladder in my small hand as tightly as I can.

On the walk home Dad abruptly decides on a detour. Instead of pushing me around the corner at 79th Street he makes a sharp left toward the garage under our building. "A change of scene," he says. The steep ramp down is dark and cool as we get closer. The descent begins, and I feel its pull beneath me. Dad holds tight to the handles of my wheelchair. The downward pressure intensifies. Before I know what's happening I'm tumbling out of my wheelchair onto the hard, oil-stained incline. And I keep rolling . . . out of control, on my own, a rag doll without enough muscle to stop myself . . . until I bump against a side wall. And just lie there.

I don't remember crying. I don't remember hurting. I remember *thinking*—having an acute, reflexive alertness to my surroundings and taking a kind of mental inventory of where I am and how I'm feeling. An out-of-body alertness. There is nothing else I *can* do. I'm too stunned to hurt or cry. I can't move anything—I *never* can—but I can be aware and wholly conscious, an omniscient observer. Then Dad is there, beside me, asking how I am, touching me, examining me for damage and scooping me up off the garage floor and placing me back in my chair. This time he remembers the seat belt.

He keeps asking if I'm okay. This is when I start to cry. A few heaves at first, then gushes. He rushes me upstairs, to our apartment, to Mom. I can't stop crying, though I try. I become breathless.

"There, there," says Mom, taking me into her arms. She quickly turns practical. "Stop your crying and tell me what hurts."

I can't stop bawling and haven't a chance of answering. She holds me still a moment and it feels warm and lovely. Then Mom sees a bump on my head. I mutter about my finger and try to produce my right hand. Its ring finger is swollen and rosy-purple and aching. Mom calls for ice, which Dad promptly delivers. My weeping subsides, replaced by a *youch* at the touch of ice to my scalp.

"You'll be fine," Mom declares.

She puts the ice to my finger and looks up at Dad with lightning bolts.

Parents of kids with disabilities tend to be unduly overprotective. It's the extra layer of guilt. From the start they feel responsible for their child's limitations. It doesn't matter if the disability is from an accident or heredity; parents see it as a gnawing reminder of their own shortcomings. They feel intrinsically blameworthy. I'm grateful my parents aren't *overly* overprotective, but they feel the guilt. For Mom, the day she learned my floppiness was permanent and inborn was the worst of her life. She tells me this whenever I ask and even when I don't. That's partly because she's concerned about my future, but she also questions what she did to deserve this. For Dad, the guilt feelings evolve into a hunt for solutions, and for someone to blame besides himself.

Many parents turn angry—an animal rage directed at doctors, bureaucrats, God, or even the child him- or herself. Sometimes these feelings spark a crusade for remediation or justice, a frantic pursuit of a lawsuit, a cure, or political action. But whatever the merits of the cause, the fire is stoked primarily by the need to alleviate the parent's unbearable burden, which is not necessarily in the child's best interest.

"You must, must, *must* remember the seat belt," Mom scolds Dad, who stands silently nodding. "How could you forget?"

A spate of rhetorical questions follows. Could she trust him ever again? By extension, if my own father can forget my seat belt what about other people to whom my care is entrusted?

"This cannot happen again!" she says repeatedly.

Then Mom's hard tone turns abruptly to me. It's in her Republican upbringing to have no patience for self-pity and whining. *Look out for yourself. Don't wait for a handout.* She's always quick with advice to *step up to the plate.* She keeps an ongoing, or quickly composed, mental to-do list, which she likes to whip out like a gunslinger.

"And Ben," she says then, "Ben, it's your responsibility to check if the person with you has forgotten your seat belt. Do you understand? Do you hear me? Ultimately it's *your* responsibility. You must always, always speak up. Understand?"

Not yet four, I'm stunned yet struggle to comprehend. I try to take her admonitions as seriously as I can. *Speak up. Don't be shy. Ask for what you need. People aren't mind readers. You've got to speak up.* I hear these phrases a lot. *Light a candle instead of cursing the darkness. The squeaky wheel, etc.*

In those days, the mid-1960s, there are scant resources for my parents to draw on, other than doctors. No support groups. No disability-rights organizations or independent-living centers. No sense of a shared, group identity disability-wise, except perhaps for disabled veterans. Any notion of the disabled as a class of ordinary citizens, a population worthy of civil rights, is years away. The first Civil Rights Act, passed in July 1964, when I'm nineteen months old—two years before my garage accident—applies almost exclusively to Black people, of course. It never occurs to anyone, let alone my parents, to extend antidiscrimination and equal opportunity to people with disabilities. Not like in the early twenty-first century, when we know that some 51 million Americans—or 18 percent of the population—have a disability, making us the single largest minority and thus unavoidably deserving of a voice supported by legislation.

The percentage of disabled Americans in the 1960s is probably smaller, though, because medicine and technology aren't yet doing such a good job of keeping us alive.

Medicine aside, to survive with a disability involves equal doses of toughness, pluck, and grit mixed with humor, a stiff upper lip, love, luck, and money. In those days, and perhaps still today, you'd best follow the Franklin Roosevelt model: Hide the handicap and its apparatus as much as possible. Minimize them. If and when they slip out, simply flash a winning grin. Use your limitation as a sign of strength and courage, not sorrow, shock, or loss. An emblem of overcoming, of achieving despite all.

But is that best?

To be sure, Mom and Dad don't exactly realize they're subscribing to the FDR model. They simply want me to remember I have nothing to fear but fear itself. Yet that afternoon, as Mom lectures me about speaking up and taking care of myself, in my mind I'm still falling down the garage ramp and smacking up against a stark reality: I'm undeniably, unavoidably vulnerable, no matter how much spunk I may possess. My new green wheelchair—a badge of growing up, of going to kindergarten, of greater independence—brings a host of unforeseen risks and burdens.

Everything is double-edged! There can be nothing good without something bad!

I'm not yet four, but I might as well be forty.

It's not right to call this premature self-awareness a kind of wisdom, though, because it's simply practical knowledge learned the hard way, an attitude derived from struggle. It's nothing to be proud of. The wisdom, if there is any, would come from knowing when to use this knowledge of vulnerability and when not to be dragged down by it. And that I have yet to learn.

Once iced, my purple finger continues to throb. It throbs for an eternity. I shy away from using my right hand to draw with. I blame myself a little for the accident. I could have remembered the seat belt.

For a month afterward Mom asks me to check my seat belt, but then she too begins to forget. She does not wallow. I want to get past it even more than she does. Over time I learn to bury, or re-bury, my frustrations and fears. I will not let bumps and barriers make me fearful or reticent. Rather, I remind myself that hardships build character. They make me a stronger person.

It's a guise I can maintain for only so long.

Perhaps even then I do have an inkling about my life ahead: I can already sense it will be split along two divergent paths—the normal expectations of a son of New York Jewish liberal educated intelligent parents to go out in the world, advance, and take charge of his own actions and fate, and the dangerous, ineluctable fragility of the hopelessly, severely disabled.

To live with this dichotomy between upwardly mobile overachiever and delicate flower with what today is foolishly called "special needs"—to live with *myself*—I'll have to learn to navigate between or, better yet, balance, redefine, and integrate these two discrepant identities and potential destinies.

It's a struggle that continues for the rest of my life.

CHAPTER TWO

DISABILITY AS A SOCIAL CONDITION

1967–1971

"The true story, as is usually the case, had a very small circulation."
—F. Scott Fitzgerald, "The Curious Case of Benjamin Button," *Tales of the Jazz Age*

I know they are discussing me, but I don't know why. I can't hear a word or see them to read body language. They have closed the door. I'm on the outside, sitting in my wheelchair between a beige sofa and a beige armchair in the mostly quiet, fluorescently lit, antiseptic waiting room. I'm nearly six years old, and I have nothing to do.

Why didn't Alec have to come, to keep me company? Not that he *would* play with me. My older brother is nothing like me. A thin, spirited boy with straight dark-reddish-brown hair and a gap between his front top teeth, he's brainy and competitive, likes to play chess and baseball and go bowling. I, on the other hand, have big blue eyes and a mop of unruly blond hair, an adorable Cupid look. Mom's friends say they wish they had my curls, which I don't understand because I hate my hair. I want it to be straight, like I see on TV.

On Saturdays Alec goes to a sports camp while I watch cartoons, and in the summer a sleepaway camp in New Hampshire while I stay home and look for ways to pass the time.

Now, in the hermetic waiting room, I imagine leaping through the big, half-sunny window, kicking past the rattling glass and landing catlike on the street below just in time to chase away a squadron of bad guys. I'd roll on the ground to avoid their gunfire and then grab a loose drainpipe or tree branch and knock them all out till the police come ... I can pass a lot of time imagining highly athletic action scenes. But alas, I soon discover it's not enough time, and my boredom resumes. I can't hold up a magazine or book, and there's no table I can get to to roll my toy cars on if I had any toy cars with me. Not that this boredom is exactly an unfamiliar phenomenon. At home, when there's no school, I complain a lot about having nothing to do. I play with my toy cars and tell myself stories until these activities bore me, too. My parents are always trying to come up with new forms of autonomous entertainment for me, beyond TV. Coloring books, cards, Etch-a-Sketch, Colorforms. If only we'd had computers then! (Perhaps this is why, in 1972, when I'm nine, we become one of the first American families to buy the Magnavox Odyssey video game console, once I demonstrate that I'm able to manipulate the controller.)

Why do I have to go to so many doctors? I wonder now.

In truth, Dr. Spiro *is* one of my favorites. Every year, before the private parent conference, he examines me and talks to me in a soft, cheerful manner. He asks me to squeeze his fingers, follow his penlight with my eyes, stick out my tongue, feel the vibrations of his tuning fork against my knees and ankles (and tell him when the vibrations stop), and perform other easy tasks to measure my muscles and nerve responses. It always seems to impress him that I'm not stone paralyzed or retarded!

I like the attention. I don't mind being on display. It's best if I can stay in my wheelchair and not get lifted onto his hard, narrow examination table and have my clothes taken off. But either way—in my chair or on his examination table, dressed or naked—I try to put on a good performance. I'm famous for my good humor and bravery. I never even cry at shots.

Finally, finally, finally the door opens and Mom and Dad come out and they're smiling and talking and shake hands with Dr. Spiro, who waves at me.

"So what was that all about?" I ask in the elevator. Dad's pushing me. I'm facing the back wall but it's a mirror so that's okay.

"Just grown-up talk," says Mom.

Mom is intense and coiled-up inside, like something forceful and beautiful wrapped in a tight package. She's about a foot shorter than Dad; Dad's a good six-feet-two-inches, with broad shoulders, though he's not athletic. One of the things Mom and Dad have in common is a great faith in doctors. To them, medical science holds all the answers. "It's not so many years since a man named Dr. Salk cured polio," Mom has told me many times.

I'm not too keen on the idea of a cure for my amyotonia, though. I'm used to my life as it is and any change would be really weird to get used to. I'm not so badly off as many people think I am. I'm not. I'm not like other handicapped kids!

In the car, my chair folded and crammed between the front and back seats, Dad driving, Mom tells me more. We always take the car to Dr. Spiro's because his office is in the Bronx or Queens or someplace like that. "Dr. Spiro is pleased with you. He feels you're doing fine."

"He always says that," I say, even though it feels good to hear.

"He sees almost no change from last year, which means your amyotonia may be stabilizing. He says it's now called spinal muscular atrophy. You're not losing strength, and you should stay the same your whole life. You know there's no cure still, but you're not getting worse."

You mean I could have been getting worse? I can't recall a time when I had more strength than I have today. I'm told I crawled a little as a baby, which I can't do now, but I figure I was smaller and lighter then. In any case, I don't remember it. I have no sense of lost capacity. So Mom's news ripples past me with little impact.

Mom says we know the worst of it now. She sounds relieved as she says this. From behind the steering wheel Dad adds, "That's good news," in case I didn't understand. If it's such good news, why was I kept out of the doctor's office? And what took so long in there? Just grownups' way of doing things, I guess. I look out the car window. It's getting dark.

If the bad guys pulled up alongside our car now and started shooting, I'd crash out through the window and jump on top of their car. I'd reach inside their window and pull out the driver. If the car started to skid off the road I'd jump off just in time. I'd roll on the ground with guns flaring. They'd run and I'd chase. They wouldn't have a chance. Even if they thought they had me they'd be proved wrong. Just when the bad guys felt I was down and out, I'd shock them by coming up strong and defeating them all, just like I surprise doctors with my strength and intelligence . . .

"Of course, you're not going to get any stronger either," Mom says then. "There are no treatments for spinal muscular atrophy, none discovered yet anyway, but that's okay, isn't it? We'll keep hoping, but meanwhile we have to get on with our lives."

I can't read her face. There's a sharp turn at the end of the Triborough Bridge. I know it's coming. It always makes me tip over sideways in my seat, and I silently brace for the inevitable.

***

I can't stand or raise my arms up high, but at this point I can use my hands pretty well. I can't cut my food but I do feed myself. I brush my teeth by mostly holding the toothbrush still and moving my mouth from side to side. I have very weak muscles, that's all. I have full sensation. My arms and legs are skeletally thin; I have scoliosis, which makes my left shoulder lower than my right, and my belly bulges because I have no abdominal muscles to hold it in. Alec sometimes calls me the Pillsbury Doughboy, poking me in my fattest ripples. It doesn't hurt much and I laugh.

I have complete control over my bathroom functions. I'll be able to father children, I'm told. And there's nothing wrong with my head, as Mom and Dad frequently point out. Dad went to Harvard; Mom's a Wellesley grad. Mental ability is important to them.

But when I get sick, it's very hard for me to cough effectively, and since asthma runs in the family there's always a lot of concern about my breathing. Normally it's fine.

I vaguely remember when Mom and I went to Johns Hopkins Hospital for my muscle biopsy, which confirmed the original diagnosis of amyotonia. I was three, and we took the train from New York. Mostly I remember being returned to Mom's arms after the surgery. I remember shivering and crying. I remember Mom's blue dress—a welcome contrast to the sickly yellows and pale greens all around—and being enwrapped in its folds. I remember confusion and fear. I remember returning home to Dad and Alec with souvenirs—a brightly-colored pinwheel and my hospital ID bracelet. Alec promptly grabbed the pinwheel from my small hand. Mom and Dad scolded him, and he dropped it onto the floor and marched around the apartment in his pajamas singing silly songs in a loud warble. Besides the pinwheel, what he stole from me was the attention. I was powerless to stop him or to retaliate.

Alec is high energy and prone to what Mom calls temper tantrums. Mom says it's because I get so much attention from her and Dad. In turn, I get Alec's attention by doing funny voices and resorting to creative name-calling. I make him laugh.

"Why are you such a freak?" I say with stealthy calm.

"Am I fr-r-r-r-eaky? Freaky! Freaky! Freaky!"

"See?"

"At least I'm not a Stu-ball, like you."

"I'm not stupid!"

But my heart isn't in it. Maybe I *am* stupid.

"I didn't say 'stupid,' Retard. But I'll bet you don't know how much sixteen times sixteen is?"

He seems so impossibly strange. So different from me. So aggressive. And probably smarter. Alec is eight and goes to a good school where he learns French and reads big books. I'm still five and can't read. I would be going to Alec's school, *L'École Française,* on the Upper East Side, but this elite institution refuses to take a kid in a wheelchair. Architectural obstacles abound, and who can predict what effect my presence may have on the other kids? It's 1968, and it's still legal to discriminate against the handicapped.

According to government statistics, only one in five handicapped kids is educated in a public school at that time—usually a separate special-ed school. The majority stays home or gets sent off to live-in institutions. More than a million handicapped kids have no access to the school system at all. Many states have statutes specifically *excluding* the deaf, blind or mentally retarded from public schooling. This despite the Elementary and Secondary Education Act of 1965, which addressed the need for equity for "educationally deprived children," as President Johnson puts it when he signs it into law. A year later the Act is amended to establish a federal Bureau of Education of the Handicapped and, under Title VI, special funding to accommodate handicapped students. This basically fueled special-ed, not inclusion or "mainstreaming" in regular schools. Not until September 26, 1973—when I'm ten years old and starting sixth grade—do handicapped kids begin to gain the right to an integrated, quality education, with passage of the US Rehabilitation Act. Its Section 504 will prohibit discrimination based on disability in educational facilities that receive federal funding. Two years later, the Education for All Handicapped Children Act will put federal money where its mouth is by supporting state efforts to improve schooling for handicapped kids. It will set no clear national standards, however, and follow-through will be slack. So fifteen years after that—in 1990, when I'm already out of college for six years—the Individuals with Disabilities Education Act will set terms for full integration in public schools of all kids with disabilities, to the fullest extent possible. Soon some six million kids with disabilities will attend public schools, receiving specialized services as needed to meet their educational requirements.

Though not held to the same standard unless they receive federal funds, private schools will gradually try, at least, to follow the example of their public counterparts.

Mom and Dad are way ahead of their time in refusing to have me segregated. In fact, they raise me in isolation from other handicapped kids. Or rather, they protect me from them. I don't want to be around other kids like me anyway, mostly because they are *not* like me. At least I don't see myself as being like them. I figure if I'm being separated from them, there's got to be a reason. There's got to be something wrong with them. They must be spastic, talk funny, and drool. I'm certain they dress badly, have choppy haircuts, and sometimes smell bad. I don't know for sure because I haven't really been around other handicapped kids, but you kind of pick up impressions.

"Handicapped" is the word my family uses—the *polite* word, that is, as opposed to "crippled."

Dad is editor of *GQ* magazine, which he calls *Gentleman's Quarterly*. Mom worked for the producers of a TV program called *Playhouse 90* on CBS before Alec was born. They're modern thinkers. In a time when it's widely accepted that even the best parents can't easily cope with having a handicapped child, or wouldn't want to, Mom and Dad go against the grain.

Yet every now and then Mom wonders if the kids who are warehoused in these special-ed ghettos develop a sense of camaraderie, of shared frustration, that I'm missing. She says being with these kids might provide me with an "emotional support system."

"Oh puh-lease!" I say.

"Don't be such a smart aleck! Sometimes people need help with emotional issues. It can't be easy being different. Being you."

"But I don't have those kinds of problems. I'm fine." *Smart aleck*, I'm thinking. Yeah, my brother Alec *is* smart. But saying anything like that will make Mom angry. Or angri*er*.

"Okay. Well, maybe talking to a psychologist sometime is something you'd like to try. Just to talk about what it's like being you. They can help you sort out your feelings and—"

"That's worse! I'm not crazy. I'm not sad. And I don't like other handicapped kids. They're gross!"

"How do you know that, dear? They might be just like you. You certainly share the problem of getting along, of confronting the non-handicapped world around you."

Confronting? "I know how to fit in." I say.

She says that's terrific and she's proud of me. For her, being properly socialized is half the point of keeping me mainstreamed. "It's important to learn to get along with others, to look nice and behave attractively, if you want to get anywhere in the world."

"*Ai-yai-yai*, Mom!"

"I don't make the rules, that's just the way it is. We all have to face it."

Mom has her reasons, beyond vanity. She grew up poor because her father, Grandpa Sam, a Cincinnati defense lawyer, had such an unpleasant manner the only clients he could keep were the most desperate and destitute.

The other reasons she and Dad insist on a regular private school are (1) they know separate isn't equal, (2) they want the best education possible for their kids, and (3) they're snobs.

So I start first grade at the Walden School, on West 88th Street. It's a regular, albeit progressive, private school with a liberal admissions policy. I mingle with kids of all colors, many on scholarships, many others from the creative elite of the Upper West Side. As the only wheelchair-riding student, I'm a pioneer of sorts. It's not exactly wheelchair accessible—each morning Dad has to schlep me, in wheelchair, up a small flight of steps at the entry, and every afternoon Mom hauls me back down again.

One evening I overhear Mom and Dad talking in the kitchen. They are grateful for Walden. Dad says he isn't sure about its prestige but Mom says it will be fine. Best of all, she says, Walden doesn't see me as a typical handicapped kid. Dad agrees. It's making an exception for me because of my intelligence and alertness, he says.

Judy, my new class teacher—a tall, slender woman with dark hair and warm eyes as expressive as a cartoon character's—quickly makes accommodations. For example, at the end of the first week she gathers the entire class of sixteen kids in a circle and introduces me. Just me! She explains why I use a wheelchair and then says something funny:

"Would any of you like to *touch* Ben's wheelchair?"

If they touch it, she explains, they won't be afraid of it. She is making a kind of case study of me for her master's thesis, it turns out, testing the concept of mainstreaming.

I'm startled to think that anyone would be afraid of my chair. Yet right away a few hands shoot up, then more. Soon I'm surrounded by grubby eager fingers. Many of these kids quickly become my new best friends. Within a day I'm appointing a trusted subset to be my first choices for wheelchair-pushing. We make a game of it—they compete to be my Chief Wheeler, and I choose the winners. "You were totally accepted by your classmates because you were so cute and so bright, just like everyone else, except you were on wheels," recalls Judy, my teacher, four decades later.

At the end of the semester she notes on my report card that I have "leadership skills." If so, it comes from necessity. It's a survival skill, a form of gentle manipulation that maybe all handicapped kids learn. Taking charge. Putting people at ease.

One kid, however, isn't so easy to figure out. On a half-cloudy November afternoon a girl named Carrie crawls across a classroom tabletop toward me, grinning. Bony and high strung, with long black hair she's always tucking behind her ears, one of many tics, she's a friend but not a member of my Club. I call my group of best friends a Club, a restricted club, and though it has no benefits other than wheelchair-pushing privileges, the other kids seem to like being members. "Hi, Ben!"

"Carrie . . . what're you doing on the table?"

She inches closer. At the edge of the table she says "hi" again. Then she's practically in my lap. She reaches out and begins unbuttoning my navy-blue corduroys and unzipping my fly—

"Carrie!" Judy yells from across the room. Carrie's white-hot face falls like a startled soufflé as she looks up and unhands my pants. Judy marches over. "Back to your seat!"

Silently, Carrie crawls away. Judy steps closer and closes my pants. No more is said about the incident. Later, when Mom comes to pick me up, Judy tells her what happened. They talk in soft voices.

On the chill walk home along Central Park West, Mom tells me to let her and Judy know if anything like this occurs again. Some children have a hard time accepting my handicap, she says. That's not so, I say, not in this case. Mom says she understands it was just play, but still. I say okay, but I'm lying. I don't want to tell Mom or Judy or anyone else if it happens again. If I commented on all the odd things people do around me, I'd never shut up.

For instance, I never tell about Quentin. He's a long-haired, pale-skinned, rangy boy with a taut, satanic grin who frightens me. It's not merely his appearance. It's something about the way he looks at me, or doesn't, with his fanatical eyes. I try ignoring him. He's one of the reasons I surround myself with a protective barrier of friends. Quentin pays us no mind, and at first I congratulate myself on a strategic victory. All goes smoothly, but only for a time.

***

To be nearer to Walden, we've moved from our second-story apartment on East 79th Street to a six-room co-op on the eighteenth floor of The Beresford, a cavernous Art Deco building on Central Park West near the Planetarium and dinosaur museum. Alec, who is eight, is against moving. He likes life to stay the same. Or maybe he just likes to argue.

Soon after moving, Mom and Dad have all the doorway thresholds removed and smoothed over, an access modification for me. This is thirty years before access modifications become codified by law. Mom and Dad and the men they hire have to figure it out on their own. Pioneers, again!

Workmen and sawdust fill the place for weeks. The light switch in the bedroom Alec and I share is lowered so I can reach it, if pushed close enough. I've never flipped a light on and off before. Who knew it was so simple? I flip it a hundred times that first day.

I remember our first Halloween there. Dad takes Alec and me trick-or-treating at our old apartment where we know people. As Dad pushes me from door to door and Alec, wrapped in crêpe paper like a mummy, follows alongside or leads the way, I never think about what I must look like in my Batman costume. A superhero who can't walk? But we do notice the unnatural attention I receive at some of the apartments we accost. At the end of the night, and pretty much every Halloween, I invariably score more loot than Alec. As if candy will cure me.

Years later, I will learn of a historical connection between Halloween and disability. I will receive ample evidence of the once-common fear of deformities—the limping, hunchbacked, hook-handed, or one-eyed monsters of ancient fairytales and old horror movies. Even the word "creepy" comes from the same word as "cripple." And when people like me weren't feared, they were often gawked at in carnival freak shows or objectified for their noble suffering . . . like Tiny Tim, whose only role in life is to inspire and cheer up other people. Mostly what I know of that objectifying comes from the medical profession, the constant stripping and prodding and X-raying and "show me your tongue"-ing I'm subjected to, ostensibly for my own good but, in truth, primarily to educate doctors about my unusual anatomy.

At school, other logistical problems quickly emerge. I start peeing in my pants. It's a logistical problem because I have no way of raising my hand to be excused, no way of taking myself to the bathroom. And I'm embarrassed to shout out for help.

"What if you had a different way to signal you need to go?" asks Mom.

She tells me to suggest a word or phrase that's easy to remember— something I wouldn't ordinarily say, which has no other meaning, and that I'll feel comfortable calling out in public. It's genius! And it's lovely because it means Mom understands.

I have no choice but to get my teacher's help in the bathroom, naturally. I don't have the luxury of privacy. Yet this should make it less humiliating. I ponder a moment.

"How about, 'Judy, one two three'?"

Mom shares the code with my teacher, who likes the idea. I tell myself I'm Jonny Quest on an adventure, complete with a secret code. Again using fantasy to deflect discomfort.

The battle may be won, but the war isn't over. In second grade I have bathroom troubles at school again. I've become too heavy for my teacher to lift onto the toilet. So one day my parents present me with a blue-green plastic jug I'm supposed to carry every day. A white canvas sack is hung on the handlebars at the back of my wheelchair. The jug fits inside, sort of. Actually, it protrudes out the top sometimes. They call it my urinal. Which doesn't make me feel any calmer in my stomach pit.

I'm afraid kids will tease me when they see it—but I must admit it should do the trick. The portable urinal is the latest step in working out the logistics of my attending a regular school, another "reasonable accommodation" my parents devise, decades before that term becomes a point of law.

But there's one more complication. This time, instead of a code, Mom sets it up for my new teacher to take me to the bathroom every day after lunch, whether I ask or not. At home I'm already going to the toilet on a set schedule, and it eases the burden of having to ask, so I accept.

It's just one example of how my life at age seven has already become highly regimented. When I'm set up at the table with crayons and paper, I know I must have everything within reach, everything I'll need for as long as possible, so I won't have to ask busy parents for extra help. They're kind, but can't always be at my beck and call. Where other seven-year-olds might choose clothes for themselves and change their minds two or three times, I'm still dressed by my parents and have to select outfits they'll accept—outfits I can stick with, too, because it's too much trouble to change my mind. There's no surprising my parents.

What's more, my entire wardrobe is memorized so I can name clothes without looking in my drawers. I'm dressed in bed, before getting to my chair, and it's impossible to see into my drawers from there.

Inevitably, a certain rigidity settles in. Spontaneity becomes a forbidden luxury, even spontaneity in peeing. My life soon feels overrun with orderliness and rationed efforts. I'm *always* required to articulate my wishes and needs, can't just act on them. I'm forced to plan ahead. And I internalize this self-discipline with near-military precision. Disability is my boot camp. Impulsiveness is drained out of me. Without realizing, I come to depend on precedent—whatever worked before should work again—because I can't trust in winging it.

***

In third grade, one of my extra special friends invites me to her apartment to play. A smart, petite girl with long, thick black hair, Joanie lives only a few blocks away. Her mom comes to escort us. Which means she's going to push my wheelchair on the sidewalk—but first, down the school steps. Joanie's mom doesn't look physically strong, yet I bravely give her instructions. I can feel her hands shake as she clutches the handlebars of my wheelchair.

One step at a time.

We get almost all the way down without incident . . . until she slips. I fly out of her hands and bound down the hard marble stairway—*k'bump-k'bump!*

I hit the bottom facedown, my chin on the lowest step, my wheelchair on top of me.

Mr. Martinez, the school's muscular and jovial maintenance man, is there, leaning over me, trying to pull me up. It's hard to talk with my chin pressed against the bottom step, but I know words are my strongest asset and best defense. Mom has drilled that into me over the years. *Speak up! People aren't mind readers!*

I manage to say, "Open the seat belt first."

The only Walden staffer not called by his first name, oddly enough, Mr. Martinez bends down to make sure he understands. I can smell his sweet cologne, and I'm grateful. It's important he understand me. If he pulls the wheelchair up without unbuckling me first, I'll twist an ankle.

He reaches under me to unfasten the belt. Released from the chair, I slide into a slightly more comfortable position on the floor. He is then able to lift me bodily—like a groom carrying his bride over the threshold—without twisting my ankle, and carry me up the steps to a sofa in the school office. Someone else brings my chair.

The school nurse looks me over, calls Mom. Joanie and her mom stay near. I'm in no pain, but the wait for Mom seems very long.

Finally she's there. The play date is canceled. No other harm done.

You become used to wheelchair accidents.

The next time Joanie and I get together it's at my apartment. By now we're considered boyfriend and girlfriend. When no one else is around, we decide to undress. So, under the pretext of needing a nap, I ask Inez, our housekeeper, to lift me out of my wheelchair and put me in bed. Once she's gone, Joanie closes the door and I instruct her how to open my jeans. She knows how, of course, but needs encouragement. "I can't unbutton them myself," I explain matter-of-factly.

She insists on going first, and begins to lower her jeans and underpants. I try to look but can't—I'm not sure what I see. Then it's my turn. To my surprise she says no. Fearing she's merely being bashful about helping me, I try my usual brand of reassurance. "You can do it. It won't hurt or anything."

I don't think about the implications of her actually touching me. We're just having fun, sharing. She continues to say no and I give up. Inez puts me back in my chair and we play ordinary board games. But it's clear: I'm not going to let my handicap get in the way of my romantic life any more than I let it detour my education or anything else.

It's a lesson I'll carry with me long into adulthood, when it really matters.

***

In 1968, the Muscular Dystrophy Association of America's Labor Day telethon is broadcast outside the New York metropolitan area for the first time. Launched in the early '50s as an occasional four-hour fundraiser on a few New York television stations, it became a nineteen-hour star-studded TV event on Labor Day 1966, though still within tight geographical boundaries. In 1969, when I'm seven, I'm invited to be the charity's head poster child.

We think highly of the MDAA (as it's known then) in my household. It tells us about my spinal muscular atrophy, what to do to keep me healthy. Mom and Dad say it helps pay for Dr. Spiro. Someday it might find a cure so I can walk, they say.

On a fall Saturday afternoon Mom takes me to a studio downtown—a large, mostly empty windowless space. At the back, under very bright lights, a quiet girl a few years older than I am stands awkwardly with the aid of crutches. She has short, dark hair and wears a short green pinafore dress that exposes leg braces. Mom says she's the outgoing model. I should speak to her for tips about what it's like to be a poster child.

I watch silently. The girl doesn't do much, just stands there as a camera clicks. Then a stout man in a dull tan suit waves for Mom to bring me over. I'm parked in my wheelchair next to the girl. An even fatter man in shirtsleeves starts snapping photos of the two of us. Am I supposed to do something? Besides squint at the bright light, that is. After a while, we're told we're done. I wonder, is this what it means to be a poster child?

The photo appears in a Sunday supplement my family doesn't normally get. I dream of fame, but no one I know sees the picture.

In December I'm photographed on Santa's lap for the *Daily News*. At seven, I'm beginning to have doubts about Santa, but I figure it's probably not the *real* one for the picture, since I'm not sure Santa does that kind of work. Some Jewish kids don't celebrate Christmas, but we do.

Two weeks later the photo appears. My parents buy a few copies of the *Daily News*, another paper they never look at. I don't pay attention to the words under the picture, but Alec tells me it says Santa cares about Jerry's kids. I have trouble understanding the phrase "Jerry's kids" because, for one thing, I've never met Jerry.

I'm invited to appear in a New York TV studio during the next Labor Day telethon, but still never meet Jerry. I meet the host of TV's *Wonderama*, Sonny Fox. And later, at another fundraising event, I meet *Wonderama*'s new MC, Bob McAllister, but that's about as exciting as it gets.

When I'm eight, I pose for a full-page magazine ad "standing" in my old uncomfortable leg braces beneath the sappy caption, "If I grow up I want to be a fireman."

If? My life expectancy is normal! Mom and Dad and Dr. Spiro have told me so.

Besides, I don't want to be a fireman. It's someone else's boyhood fantasy, someone who can walk and climb, perhaps, but not mine. I want to go further; I want to be a superhero, a police detective, a starship captain, a brilliant scientist like Dr. Quest on *Jonny Quest,* but never a fireman.

I keep my fingers crossed behind my back as the camera clicks. I look up, visualize a secret laboratory and sparkling, computerized panels in an attempt to communicate my true desires by ESP. Afterward I tell Mom I want to quit being a poster child. She asks if I'm sure but offers no further objection.

The truth is, I'm beginning to recognize that I'm not particularly interested in being able to walk. I've invested a lot in getting used to life on wheels. I like having someone always with me, pushing me and protecting me from the world. Walking seems a dangerous way to get around, two legs a perilous perch. Aren't walkers always complaining about sore and tired feet? Being in a wheelchair is part of what makes me stand out from the crowd, so to speak. It's a piece of my identity.

My "identity" seems to be one thing in these MDA ads and quite another in my real-world daily life. My handicap may be measurable to Dr. Spiro, but what it means—its impact on who I am and my place in the world—is open to broad interpretation.

The following Labor Day, after I've quit, we turn on the TV to watch a little bit of the telethon. To me, it's boring and corny and my mind wanders. Mom doesn't like TV (which is funny since she used to work in TV), and has little patience for the broadcast despite her fondness for the muscular-dystrophy organization itself, but Dad is transfixed. "Oh, oh, oh!" he erupts suddenly with forced melodrama. "Those poor kids! I've got to call right now and pour out my nickels and dimes!"

Then he bursts into a hearty laugh. Alec laughs at Dad's laughing, and I do too. I'm not sure I get the joke, but it has something to do with the schmaltzy profiles of weird, dying kids. Usually Alec and I like to watch comedies like

F Troop and *I Dream of Jeannie*, which Mom and Dad don't watch with us. Another show I like is *Ironside*, which Mom suggested I try. She thinks I like it because the police chief is in a wheelchair, but that's not really the point of the show, is it? Still, it's a very different image of people like me than what you usually see on the telethon.

"You shouldn't make fun of them," Mom says, reentering the room. The TV is in Mom and Dad's bedroom, and she's come in to get something from her desk. "Just because they're not like Ben doesn't give you the right. It's a good cause and it just might help Ben one of these days."

Dad says he's sorry and didn't mean any harm. "I know it's important," he says from the phone. He's gotten up from their king-size bed to call in a donation. *They're not like Ben.* That's what Mom said. That's what I hear. It's been the going line for a long time. I'm different from other handicapped kids. When people treat me like I *am* one of those pathetic dying kids, when strangers feel sorry for me, it's funny in both senses of the word—odd and humorous. On occasion little old ladies offer to buy me cookies, and my parents won't let them. Mom says I shouldn't feel sorry for myself and shouldn't encourage other people to either.

So why, I wonder, does she defend the telethon? It does bring images of kids in wheelchairs into people's homes, instead of maintaining the status quo of unsightliness and shame. But it certainly doesn't make them look good or competent or equal. It doesn't glamorize them. It offers them up covered in a syrupy goo of sentimentality.

And if those kids aren't like me—and they aren't—then why does Mom say the Muscular Dystrophy Association helps families like ours? What's it got to do with me? I don't have muscular dystrophy. I'm not going to die from my spinal muscular atrophy—that's what Dr. Spiro says, anyway. I've outlived the dying phase.

I don't see how the pathetic spazzes on the telethon have anything to do with me except for being in wheelchairs.

Unless I'm wrong about myself. About them.

No, I definitely don't want to be confused with those kids. I don't want to feel sorry for them, either. It's too depressing to bear, and I wonder if it's real anyway, if those kids are as bad off as they say, or if they're actually like me and the telethon is just telling people to feel sorry for them. In any case, I'm brought up to keep moving forward, never to pause for pity. Pity is useless, the enemy of self-esteem and industry.

Mom always says I can be anything I want when I grow up, and I believe it's true.

CHAPTER THREE

DIVORCE, BAR MITZVAHS, AND PREADOLESCENCE— WASN'T MY LIFE HARD ENOUGH?

1972–1976

> "For her, of course, the measure of how you held up in the face of a life-threatening illness was not how much you changed but how much you stayed the same, in control of your own identity."
>
> —Calvin Trillin, *About Alice*

Over Thanksgiving weekend back in 1955, my parents meet. It's a blind date set up by Dad's Aunt Clara. Dad—then just Everett—is twenty-seven, visiting home (Columbus, Ohio) from Los Angeles, where he's been the past five years, since graduating magna cum laude and Phi Beta Kappa from Harvard. He's earning a master's in English at UCLA and working as a sales clerk at the May Company on Wilshire Boulevard, among other odd jobs. He has considered law school for next year, yet finds the reading list intimidating. In truth, he isn't at all sure what to do with the rest of his life. He's also grown tired of LA's beautiful but, alas, intellectually mediocre women.

He ventures to Paula's Cincinnati home—a tidy, cramped, two-room row house—with some trepidation. Paula, just nineteen, is home from Wellesley College, where she's a junior. An only child from a poor family. What could they possibly have in common?

After shaking hands, Paula's father immediately washes his right hand. He's an odd bird with a kind-eyed but brittle-looking wife, who doesn't want to let Paula go when it's time to leave.

Paula, petite and pretty in an unconventional way—not *too* pretty, thankfully!—seems eager to hightail it. She wears her shoulder-length wavy brown hair in a modern, unfussy way, and owlish black-rimmed glasses.

At the candle-lit restaurant, chosen on the authority of Aunt Clara, their conversation moves quickly to literature and art and philosophy . . . his passion for Lionel Trilling . . . hers for Joyce . . . his chauvinism for Dickens, Thomas Mann, and the masterful E. M. Forster . . . hers for Graham Greene and Maupassant . . . the influence of Benjamin Disraeli and the rise of Jewish secularism . . . and the pleasures of European cinema, especially Renoir's *La Grande Illusion* and De Sica's *Bicycle Thief* and a rising Swedish director named Ingmar Bergman. He's beguiled by her academic curiosity—her very vocabulary!—and even her enthusiasm for Tom Lehrer. So different from the empty chatter of LA girls.

Three weeks later they set a wedding date—December 27, which will be Paula's twentieth birthday. Yet a few days before the wedding, Mrs. Plotnick confronts Everett. "If you're having second thoughts, say so now. Hurt my daughter *before* the wedding, not after."

It's uncanny! Has Everett let slip that he's feeling too young to be sure of anything, let alone love, and thinking Paula, though poised and self-confident, is practically a child who couldn't know what she's doing? "Don't be silly," he says.

"Come now. You can tell *me*. If you don't want to face Paula directly. Be a mensch."

But isn't a mensch *supposed* to be married, certainly by his age? It's the right thing to do. After all, to put his cold feet in perspective, he's never sure of anything.

In retrospect, their intellectual compatibility notwithstanding, their backgrounds are substantially different. Everett's family is well-to-do. His father, Jacob—whom he finds a contemptible, intimidating, Old Country boor—is a shrewd businessman. Arriving at Ellis Island at age twelve all alone, in steerage from Russia by way of England, Jacob Mattlin made his way to Columbus with nothing. He had distant family there who provided scant help, only a geographical destination.

Once settled in Columbus, Jacob Mattlin launched a successful cooperage. He made pickle barrels for the H. J. Heinz Company; other customers may or may not have included bootleggers. Jack, as he became known, married a beautiful American woman—the daughter of a previous generation of Russian immigrants, who had grown up in the neighboring state of Kentucky—and they had two sons. When Irwin, the younger one, died at the tender age of nine from influenza, Jack and Jennie went and had another. They named the replacement boy Everett—a goyish appellation, connoting their assimilation.

The Great Depression, and possibly the repeal of Prohibition, nearly wiped out Jack's barrel business, but the scrappy entrepreneur pulled himself up again by launching a machine shop that supplied the war effort (Everett was shocked to discover his father paid off officials, in whiskey, not to inspect the factory's quality control too closely) and buying property cheap.

The legend goes on and on. Everett's never sure how much of it's true, but he never could live up to his larger-than-life papa. Unlike his brother Morey—sixteen years his senior—who would've played football at Ohio State, if not for his "trick knees" (caused by a baseball injury in high school!), and served as a private in World War II (though he never went overseas, thanks to a deal Jack worked out with the local congressman), and would soon inherit and expand the family real-estate business.

For the bookish Everett, having a child with a disability years later is maybe another sign of failing to live up to some standard.

By contrast, Paula's nebbishy father, Samuel Plotnick, the germ-obsessed struggling attorney, born in Ohio to immigrant parents from Lithuania, was unyieldingly pious. His wife, the former Molly Bernhardt, of Baltimore, who emigrated as an infant with her family from Latvia, maintained an Old World stoicism. What was the use in complaining about her husband's religious strictures or the miserable, hardhanded life he made for them? This became her way in all things.

When as a small child Paula tripped and scraped her knees, Molly told her not to cry. "Scrapes are a fact of life. Scabby knees mean you're having fun! Now pull your socks up before your father comes home from shul."

The message was clear: Feeling sorry for yourself does no good. Years later, Paula will revert to this lemonade-from-lemons coping mechanism in reaction to my disability.

Given all their differences, perhaps it's not surprising my parents' marriage dissolves after seventeen years. It's 1972—practically everybody is divorcing! I'm nine years old, Alec is twelve. Dad, forty-four, is doubtless in the midst of a midlife crisis. Yet could my disability—the strain it puts on them, the differences in their reactions to it—be partly responsible?

Before I'm born—before Alec, for that matter—Dad quits teaching freshman composition at Boston University to take the editorship of a new quarterly magazine called *Apparel Arts*, later renamed *Gentleman's Quarterly*, or *GQ*. The young couple moves to New York's Upper East Side. Paula lands a job at CBS television, where she works alongside celebrities John Houseman, John Frankenheimer, and others. Richard Burton propositions her while she's pregnant with her first child (she turns him down), who will be named Jay Alexander—"Jay" after his late grandfather Jacob/Jack, though the family always calls him Alec.

When Paula, then twenty-five, brings her beautiful, brown-haired baby to Cincinnati to show her parents, she's greeted with faint half-smiles. "Don't you want to hold your *first* grandson?"

Molly has been having pains she won't talk about. With infant in tow, Paula has to drive her mother to the hospital; Sam won't go near the germ-ridden place or spend the money for gas, and Molly never had a driver's license.

She's diagnosed with ovarian cancer. Oh Lord! One of the deadliest forms, says the doctor, and highly hereditary! Within months, Molly, barely fifty, is dead. An indelible foreshadowing haunts my mother the rest of her days.

When I'm born, two and a half years later—an adorable round head and sad blue eyes, with reed-thin arms and legs—I'm given the middle name Michael and Hebrew name *Melech* after Molly. "Benjamin" is after the obstetrician.

***

The windy, early-spring night they tell us they're splitting, after an oddly solemn dinner, Alec and I fall silent, not comprehending. Then Alec is full of questions. Where will Dad go? Who will tell us stories now? Will we still get presents on birthdays?

I'm too confused for questions and stay quiet, absorbing. Let Alec do the spluttering. Until I start crying and Mom takes me on her lap. "Isn't my life hard enough already?" I say.

My words steal my parents' attention from Alec, with all his questions. Doubtless one of my goals. I've never spoken such words of self-pity before. To my mind, it's a ploy. If I push that button, play that card, I can make them take back this idiotic separation idea. Perhaps I can hurt them in the bargain, just like they're hurting us.

Mom holds me tighter. Dad wails and pats my curly head. And I see the power of words—of *my* words.

Whether or not I want to admit it, I also intend Mom and Dad to know that despite my well-adjusted cheerful exterior I do have frustrations even they can't resolve. It's not politically correct anymore to blame our bodies' limitations for our woes. It's better—more accurate and more constructive—to hold accountable the "oppressors": the vast, unaccepting "majority culture" of the able-bodied. Yet at some basic level people with disabilities do struggle against their own bodies. That may seem self-evident, but many in the then-burgeoning disability-rights movement minimize these frustrations. They fail to acknowledge the obvious— that no amount of societal attitude adjustment or legislated access will ever solve all the difficulties. Some of the struggle is inborn, like it or not, and unsolvable.

Why any of this would make any difference to Mom and Dad's marital situation, I can't say. It surprises me, but they never forget my simple, sorrowful statement. It's repeated back to me over the years. Besides the power of language, I learn that using other people's sympathy can be a formidable tool. My secret weapon. That evening, the power frightens me a little, but I like the melty feeling as Mom rocks me on her lap and Dad pats me.

In the weeks and months afterward, I regret drawing attention to my pitifulness. So I revert to type—moderately cheerful, humorously cynical, heroic.

Outwardly, my parents' separation hits Alec harder than me. He doesn't take to Dad's new lady friend, Barbara. The Sunday after his bar mitzvah, Alec throws a knock-down-drag-out tantrum when Dad decides he has to go to Barbara's niece's First Communion, on Long Island, instead of taking us to Adventureland. "But it's my bar mitzvah weekend!" Alec keeps saying.

I go with Dad. I like Barbara. Alec stays home with Mom, who cancels her own plans for his sake.

As for Barbara, part of Alec's problem might be that Dad introduced me to her first. Only about three weeks into the separation, on a sticky, sweltering

Saturday in late June while Alec's away at sleepaway camp, Dad takes me to Coney Island, and she's there—tall and thin in a yellow T-shirt and blue-jeans skirt that shows her knees, with long straight brown hair that hangs down like drapes, unadorned, on either side of her head, no makeup, and round glasses. Very 1972. She's twenty-six, a dozen years younger than Mom and nearly nineteen years younger than Dad.

Dad presents her coyly, "my friend from the office." I like her right away, not realizing her part in all that's going on.

Late in the afternoon I ask where she lives. Dad grins. "Can't you guess? Isn't it obvious?" It isn't, to me. "With *me*," he continues. "We're sharing an apartment in Brooklyn." I confess to a confused sensation of shock and betrayal. A joke? I wonder.

Do I resent what's going on? Am I angry at Dad for upending our lives? I'm too young, too accepting, to question let alone take umbrage. Yet the fracturing—and simultaneous expansion—of my world, my sense of family, will have repercussions on my psyche, my feelings about commitment and flexibility, about liberty versus stability and comfort.

Gradually my disbelief turns to fascination, especially when I visit their brownstone. I've never been in a brownstone before. Dad has to take me up two flights of steps.

Sure, Barbara's different from other adults Alec and I are used to. She's a lapsed Catholic, for one thing. Which is not necessarily bad. Later that year we have our first real Christmas tree! (We'd had Santa before, but never a tree.)

For me, the biggest adjustment is I no longer have Dad to wash and dress me every morning. He only takes care of me on alternate weekends and holidays. Mom tries to fill in but soon finds the task too onerous. So my parents join forces to hire babysitter types—mostly scary-exotic women from the Islands, who talk different. To Alec and me, they are foreign invaders, and we're shockingly intolerant, though I think primarily we're just not happy about having new hired help of any kind. Evenings and weekends, when they're gone, Alec does a hilarious imitation of fat Ena, who's from Trinidad: He waddles around our apartment muttering about "De Ba-bull! De Ba-bull!"

Ena is succeeded by Elizabeth, from Guyana, who hates winter. "Oh Behn! I's col' ou'side. So col' col' col'," I mimic to Alec's paroxysms of wheezy laughter.

It's terrible, in retrospect. I wouldn't want people making fun of *me* for how I look or sound different from others. But in our prepubescence, the humor flows freely and is a welcome release. It works off the stress of having these new people around.

Relying on hired helpers is a difficult transformation, but it'll prove key to my achieving a greater degree of independence. The whole idea of *dependent* autonomy, of being self-directed by relying on others, is a new concept that activists in Berkeley, California, are promulgating. I don't know about that at the time, yet on some level I know learning to manage my own assistants will ultimately enable me to grow up.

And marginalizing Dad from my daily life—distancing myself from his inability to accept the permanence of my disability, his hunger to uncover a cure—becomes liberating, too. I express and mask my mixed feelings towards him with a little song I make up. "Oh, my daddy, so sweet and so plump"— which he never was—"he looks like a camel without a hump!" It always makes Alec laugh, and Dad tolerates it. No one ever realizes the hostility behind it.

In the end, I decide the divorce isn't a tragic turn but a fortuitous one, because it sets me free. Yet the ghosts of my parents' breakup—the encroaching sense of familial bonds as stifling, strangling—will haunt me.

***

That same year, 1972, the nation's first curb ramp for wheelchairs is cut at the corner of Bancroft Way and Telegraph Avenue in Berkeley—the result of lobbying from a recently established group called the Center for Independent Living. The CIL is launched by a small cadre of physically disabled activists, mostly graduates of the University of California at Berkeley, with a mission to give people with disabilities the means to control their own lives, have full and equal access to everything society has to offer, and live outside of institutions, in their own homes, with the assistance of personal aides they hire and control themselves.

This is very different from any sense of what it means to be handicapped that I've ever known. It's antipodal to Dad's view of it as a mark of failure, a problem to be solved, or Mom's semi-stoic proclivity to just cope and get on with the business at hand, fighting misery with industry.

It's different from my own formulation, at ten, that disability can be ignored if you've got enough character, intelligence, and humor to rise above it.

The independent-living "model" is nothing short of revolutionary.

Spearheading this revolution is a visionary named Edward V. Roberts, who will become known as the father of the modern disability-rights movement. Nineteen years earlier, in 1953, at the age of fourteen, Roberts contracted polio and found himself unable to move, in a hospital bed, using an iron lung (portable ventilators hadn't been invented yet). There, he made a discovery similar to the one I'm making in the early '70s—the discovery of a new kind of freedom.

Here's how Ed Roberts describes it years later:

> I decided that I wanted to die. I was fourteen years old. Now, it's very hard to kill yourself in a hospital with everything set up to save your life. But the mind is a powerful thing. I stopped eating. They started to force feed me. It was really demeaning. I dropped to fifty-four pounds.
>
> My last special duty nurse left, and the next day I decided I wanted to live. You see, that was a big turning point. Up until then, these nurses were available and doing things for me around the clock—I didn't have to make any decisions for myself because they were always there. When they all finally left, that's when I realized that I could have a life, despite what everyone was saying. I could make choices, and that is freedom. I started to eat again.

Roberts and his crew, who call themselves the Rolling Quads, are fighting against a system in which institutionalization of the disabled is still widespread. Some states go so far as to forcibly sterilize people with certain disabilities. Some prohibit marriage for the genetically disabled, for fear of procreating hereditary conditions like mine. Visibly disabled people are actually barred from appearing in public in cities such as Columbus, Ohio—Dad's hometown—until 1972, and Chicago until 1974, under what are collectively called the "ugly" laws because they target anyone perceived as unattractive, for being a disturbance of the peace.

The movement to change all this and more is rising in discrete pockets all over, inspired by Black civil rights.

Closer to home, in New York City, at the very same time though unbeknownst to me, Judith Heumann organizes a group called Disabled in Action to push for equal-access legislation. If Ed Roberts is the father of disability rights, Judy Heumann is the mother. She, too, is a polio survivor and wheelchair-user. In the 1950s she went to court to win the right to attend New York public schools, and in the '60s sued for the right to teach in them.

But I'm not aware of any of this at the time. I have nothing to do with other handicapped people because the only ones I've seen are the kids on the Jerry Lewis telethon or in the special schools or summer camps I'm sometimes threatened with having to attend—the ones who are treated patronizingly, as if they haven't a brain in their heads. I know I'm not like those kids, so I think I have nothing in common with any other people who have disabilities. ("Disabilities" is already becoming the correct word in some circles, but not mine. I'm still *handicapped*.)

I'm ignorant that others are making or have made the same sorts of discoveries I'm struggling with. Feeling alone in my struggle, I become unsure of myself, unsure of whether I'm moving forward or backward. At ten, I'm increasingly conscious of my physical limitations. I may even be growing slightly weaker, though it's not obvious except I don't seem to be burning calories as effectively as I used to. I gain fifty pounds between annual doctor visits. I have to buy clothes measured in "husky" sizes. With my hopelessly curly, sandy-colored hair, I look more like a sybarite Bacchus than an angelic Cupid—though whether my fatness is a cause or an effect of my growing insecurity I won't hazard to guess. Maybe my parents' split-up is a contributing factor.

I begin emulating Chief Ironside's grouchy, hard-boiled demeanor from TV, if not his girth. Not a pretty combination—the softness on the outside propping an ineffective pillow against a molten hardening within.

***

A new medical problem further sours the mix. My scoliosis worsens, and my atrophying muscles become less effective at holding my spine in anything resembling a straight line. I have to start wearing an uncomfortable back brace—a tailor-made contraption of hard metal and pliant, aromatic leather and other industrial materials. It sticks up around my left shoulder—which as I said is lower than the right one, that being the nut of the problem—making it partially visible under my shirt. It also pinches me painfully under the arm and on one side of my waist, turning patches of skin red and raw.

The brace maker, a tall Geppetto of a man who wears a dust-colored apron and has a graying, bushy mustache, explains the chafing is caused by the brace's riding up in the course of the day. At least I think that's what he says. He mumbles with a European accent of indeterminate origin.

Mr. Snuffles, as I secretly call him, has a musty workshop on the second floor of a walk-up on the Upper East Side. Dad has to carry me bodily up the stairs. Once there, Dad lies me down on a vinyl-topped examination table, where I have nothing to do but stare at an assortment of fliers posted on the wall.

"Four out of five dentists surveyed recommend sugarless gum for their patients who chew gum" one of the signs informs me. I wonder what it's doing in a prosthetics and orthotics facility.

Decades later I will learn that the earliest recorded example of a prosthesis is an iron leg made for one Queen Vishpla, an Indian warrior in 3000 BC, who was amputated in battle yet returned to fight again with her new hardware, according to an ancient Sanskrit text.

Why isn't something like that—emboldening info about the historical importance of assistive technology—posted here? I'd much prefer a handicapped warrior to the clichéd dental-hygiene tidbit whose only relevance is a pseudo-medical connection!

Then Mr. Snuffles returns with my brace, to which he's affixed two straps. "Zey go here, you shee? *Shniff*. . .," he chatters as he snaps the new straps around either side of my groin.

Within a few days my crotch becomes redder and rawer than my waist and armpit ever did. A few weeks later, my parents agree to remove the straps. Another torture device the medical geniuses think up gets the heave-ho, though of course I have to keep wearing the brace, pinchy and irritating as it is.

I never complain about the brace at school. Doing so might incur pity. I pretend it isn't there, but I'm becoming ineluctably resentful of other people's freedom of movement.

In sixth grade, when I turn eleven, Quentin threatens to push my chair down the stairs for no discernible reason. The long-haired boy who's frightened me since first grade, he still has the beady eyes that never take me in whole. We're alone in the hallway; I told my friend Adam to go ahead, not to be late for his class, because I'm confident someone else will come along for me. Quentin happens to be the first person who does.

"I could push you right down those steps, and you couldn't stop me," he says coolly, between heavy breaths. "No, really, nothing you could do, is there? If I wanted to. And I think I do—"

"You won't," I answer, though I believe he's entirely capable of acting on his minatory words. "You know I'll tell and you'll be in deep shit."

"I'll say it was an accident."

"I can make people believe me."

"But you can't stop me. You can't do anything about it!"

He's got me there. And the more he says it, the more my insides shake. Not my outsides. I won't give him the satisfaction. "You're not going to do it. It'd be stupid."

It *would* be stupid. At best he'd get kicked out of school. If I got really hurt he could be put in jail. At least that's the way I'm thinking. Can I convince him?

It becomes a staring contest. For strength, I think about Captain Kirk in "The Corbomite Maneuver." It's all about the bluff.

Then, just as abruptly as he appeared, Quentin turns and walks away, giggling under his breath. When he's far enough I close my eyes and count to ten. I have enough time to calm down before a teacher shows up and pushes me to my classroom. I don't tell her or anyone else. Don't want to portray my fear and potential vulnerability, or incur Quentin's retribution. Yet I feel good. I think of the Winston Churchill quote, one of many Dad cites on occasion: "Nothing in life is so exhilarating as to be shot at without result."

All goes smoothly for a time. Then, a year later, when I'm twelve, I vent my frustrations on a good friend named Randy. Randy and I like to play *Ironside*, or at least I do. He's always Mark because, well, he's Black. (Guess whom I play?) On the show, Mark is the street-smart dude who drives the chief everywhere and helps him at home while attending law school. I actually like Mark better than the other supporting characters, so Randy has a position of honor. I don't think of it as racial stereotyping. In fact, sometimes secretly I wish I *were* Black; the minority status resonates with me.

We play *Ironside* at school, and we play *Ironside* at my apartment. My building's labyrinthine basement is a great place to let your imagination run wild. Plus I have a new motorized wheelchair—my first. It's too heavy to get up the school steps, but at home I love to zoom around. In my basement, Randy and I are always careful to stay clear of the housekeepers who do laundry and the maintenance workers' office as we explore the myriad dark passages and commodious storage lockers, pretending we're on a mystery investigation. It's taken me a while to get an electric wheelchair. They've been mass-produced since 1956, when Everest and Jennings rolled the first one out of its California factories, improving upon designs putatively sketched by George Westinghouse in the late-nineteenth century and British engineers during the first World War, then perfected in the early '50s by a Canadian inventor named George Klein, primarily for World War II vets—demonstrating the connection between war and disability progress.

The first E & J power chairs were notoriously slow, but in the early '70s they become the vehicle of choice for active quadriplegics—brandished by Ed Roberts and his trendsetting crew in Berkeley. The only reason I didn't have one before is Dr. Spiro feared it'd make me lazy, make me not use my arms and build strength. Now we know I can't "build up" my muscles; they will remain the way they are no matter what I do, so he finally wrote the prescription.

The first day I got the motorized wheelchair home I chased Alec all around the apartment. I wasn't a good driver yet and kept crashing, leaving tell-tale gray scratches on the white walls.

One afternoon at school, Randy spills paint on a picture I'm drawing. Maybe it was an accident. Maybe he had a good reason. The unforgivable point is his bravado about my defenselessness. "How are *you* going to get me?" he taunts.

I'll make him sorry for that. I can't fight him physically, but I have other powers. Remember? Words and sympathy are my raw tools.

I look around the classroom. Everyone's gone to PE. I'm excused and Randy is too, to keep me company. If he resents being my companion, he never says so.

Slowly, silently, I start dumping books and papers and pencils out of my small desk. I have just enough arm strength to reach in and move things out. Gradually, one by one, I cover the entire floor within a two-food radius of where I'm sitting. Some of the papers sail even farther—which I was counting on. Randy watches in disbelief.

When the other kids and Ray, our teacher, return, I don't have to say a word. Someone immediately notices the shambles and demands to know what happened. "Randy threw my stuff all over the floor," I allege.

Randy stares in shocked betrayal, tears welling in his eyes. "No I didn't."

Our teacher doesn't say a word. He's in a spot. Accuse the handicapped boy or the Black boy? I feel no regret. I am ... proud. I've mastered the perks of disability.

A girl in our class says, "How could Ben throw so far?" And I know I've won. Never mind that in trying to prove I'm not helpless I've actually reinforced the opposite—made people think Randy took advantage of me.

Even after Ray asks the class to help clean up, I stay mum. This new course I'm on—aggressive, spiteful—satisfies my insecurities. If Randy had gotten in big trouble, perhaps I would've broken. I would've relented. He doesn't, which may mean our teacher suspects. Doesn't matter. Randy's an innocent victim of my need to flex my meager power, but I figure you have to be tough to survive in a sometimes unfriendly world.

Sure, I'm fat and wear glasses and a weird-looking back brace, and have a stupid green jug urinal sticking out of the bag on my back—but I still have inner strength. I may be easily pushed in my wheelchair, but I won't be pushed around. So I willfully resolve to remain truculent ... preemptively thick-skinned and bristly ... until, in time, another discovery prompts a counter-pledge.

***

In 1975, when I'm in eighth grade, Congress passes the Education for All Handicapped Children Act, mandating full integration of kids like me in regular public schools. It's historic, but if my parents are aware of it they don't tell me—or if they do, it doesn't register.

That same year California Governor Jerry Brown names Berkeley's Ed Roberts to be director of the sunshine state's Rehabilitation Department, the first time a former claimant of government largesse has risen to such a position. I say "claimant," and not "recipient," for a good reason. As a student, Roberts was turned down for educational/vocational assistance because he was deemed unemployable. Now he'll forever alter the criteria for evaluating the potential of people with disabilities.

I haven't heard of Ed Roberts yet, but Mom does tell me about a man in Ireland who is so paralyzed he paints with his left foot. She says he's written a book about it. I'm not looking for role models of people with disabilities, and I can't understand why she tells me these things. She's still concerned that I might need some emotional bolstering due to being handicapped, even though I've already done so much, gotten so far, and scarcely ever felt sorry for myself.

Shortly after my bar mitzvah—celebrated with a buffet of my favorite foods, in the ballroom of the reform temple two-and-a-half blocks from our apartment—Mom says, "It's time you had a man's help."

Help with what? I wonder. And why a man? Ah, she means instead of the Caribbean women we like to make so much fun of. I'm embarrassed. Does she think there's something . . . inappropriate . . . going on with them? "For your privacy," she clarifies.

Privacy isn't something I'm especially concerned about. I've been naked in front of almost every adult I've ever known!

The first man we hire is a counselor at a day camp I attend the next summer. It's a handicapped camp on Long Island, which I've consented to since it's the only kind of camp that'll take me and I'm tired of being bored every summer while Alec goes off to sleepaway camp in the woods of New England. It's my first protracted experience among . . . *them.*

I try not to stare at how some sit in their wheelchairs stooped over or twisted sideways—or how their legs splay open on either side when they lie supine to get changed into bathing suits. I hope to God I don't look *that* handicapped, though I fear my prayer is hopeless. At fourteen, I regard my disability chiefly as a matter of vanity.

Austin is the best and most popular counselor, able to lift any one of us easily and swing us around for fun. He always shares his pretzels at lunch, tells us he won't go to Vietnam if drafted because he's adamantly nonviolent, and claims to rush home every afternoon to rescue the bugs in his family's inflatable pool. I want to move in with him and his family. When Mom asks if there are any counselors I'd like to have as my helper in August, it's an easy choice.

We have a small house on Fire Island. Austin stays in the guest bedroom. Once I overhear Mom talking with her friends; all the women have a crush on him.

In the fall Austin attends Yeshiva University. Soon he introduces me to Orthodox Judaism. It's alien, so different from the Reform version I've known, but I love the structure, the myriad rules (and loopholes!) for every aspect of life. No need to chart your own course. And I think this may be the answer to my confusion and self-doubt—to the bewilderment brought on by divorcing parents, budding sexuality, and being grievously disabled in an overachiever milieu. "I want to keep kosher," I declare to Mom one day.

She's harried, post-separation. She's been looking for work, getting only short stints here and there. She's furious at Dad for abandoning her, for finding new love when she can't, or won't, and for looking so good in his forties. *Why do men get better looking while woman fall apart?*, I've heard her ask no one in particular. I don't realize my turning kosher will make more work for her, cost more money. But she knows exactly what's involved, even though she hasn't kept kosher since Grandpa Sam died, when I was about five.

Needless to say, Mom is less than thrilled. Yet she goes along. As a compromise, she buys me a glass plate. We're pretty sure glass is nonporous and so can be used for both meat and dairy (though not, of course, at the same time or within three to six hours of each other).

I thrive on the rational authority of the six-hundred-and-thirteen commandments. I get Alec to go along, to a degree. On Friday afternoons, before Shabbat, he pre-tears toilet paper and loosens the refrigerator lightbulb so it doesn't turn on when opened. I can't actually tear my own toilet paper or open the refrigerator, but it wouldn't be right to have someone else break halachic code for me! We set timers to turn lights and the TV on and off during Shabbat—there's a new Saturday morning *Star Trek* cartoon I can't miss—and give up Chips Ahoy cookies for pareve Stella D'oros. I stop driving my electric wheelchair on Saturdays and, though I'm rarely up for going to synagogue, I start wearing tzitzit and a yarmulke everywhere.

"What is this crap?" is Dad's reaction. He smiles after he says it, but Dad is a modern, intellectual Jew who prides himself on getting away from "all that atavistic, Old World nonsense." You should hear him on the Hasidim! "Do they want to go back to the Dark Ages?" Barbara, who's Catholic, has a hard time with the minutiae but she's had her own bouts of religious zealotry and is less antagonistic. In college (which was only about five years ago) she even contemplated becoming a nun.

To my parents, it may be only an "adolescent phase," but for me Orthodoxy's rigidity is directly linked to my own strict life. I derive strength from the clear-cut, unwavering severity, which I'm accustomed to from my disability. Planning and intellect over emotional whim and spontaneity. Brain over body.

One glorious release from this rigidity, so to speak, is masturbation. Whether kosher or not, I indulge nightly. I have zero privacy but try to keep it secret. One midsummer weekend I go with Dad and Barbara to the Jersey Shore, where I eat nothing but fried fillet of sole—fish because I believe it fits kashruth, and fried sole because that's the only fish dish I can stand. While pushing my manual wheelchair on a quiet path, having left Barbara behind at the motel pool, Dad says, "Tell me, Ben, are you able to . . . reach yourself?"

It takes a moment to understand. I resist the giggles. Really, I'm delighted. So nobody's caught on?

Here's how I've been keeping my nightly ejaculations private and undetected: First, I ask to sleep on my back, though I can't actually sleep that way. I ask to have my hands laid flat on either thigh. I say it's more comfortable that way. Then I say goodnight and the light's turned out, the door partially closed. I have just enough hand strength to do what I need . . . After, I wait for the spew to dry before calling out to roll over.

"Yes. No problem there," I'm saying as Dad rounds a turn. The Jersey Shore is a sexy place. Lots of skin, and a certain casual attitude. My imagination gets a little carried away. "Now, Dad," I say, "can I ask *you* something?"

"Fair enough."

"What would you do if I said no, I can't?"

Of course, I'm hoping he was going to offer a prostitute to break me in. A warm breeze blows and seagulls caw. Dad laughs. "It's a good question!"

***

On the long car ride home, Dad asks me trivia questions to pass the time. Literature. World capitals. History. Simple math. I'm a disaster! No, Spain is not the capital of Italy! Boy do I get shit for that blunder. I haven't read the books Alec has, haven't studied the subjects. Blame my weird school. Or maybe I am just dumber. So as soon as I'm home I tell Mom I want to transfer for high school. She consults by phone with Dad a few days later, and in the end they don't argue with me. They've seen the problems at Walden.

When it comes to equal access, we learn, schools haven't changed much. It's 1976, and the Education for All Handicapped Children Act has been on the books only a few months. The new law harks back to a 1972 court decision in *Mills v. Board of Education*. Not as famous as *Brown*, but similarly significant for the disabled. Basically, the court ruled that the District of Columbia could not exclude children with disabilities from the public schools.

Nevertheless, here in Manhattan, the old barriers and prejudices remain. Excuses are made—Walden is famous for not giving letter grades, only teachers' comments, leaving other high schools free to claim they have no basis for evaluating my abilities. I begin to doubt them myself. Watching preppy kids lug heavy books through the cavernous corridors of Dalton School on the Upper East Side, for instance—Dad foots the bills for our education; he complains about money but always seems to have it, and when Alec and I ask him years later how he afforded private schools on an editor's salary, he merely shrugs and says he doesn't know—and talking about requirements and prerequisites with administrators who look like librarians in their cardigans and bifocals (the teachers are a bit scruffier), I begin to fear I'm too far behind to function at a "better" school.

Mom sends me to an education guidance counselor, who evaluates my skills and recommends a small school on the Upper East Side called Rudolf Steiner. Time passes, but ultimately I'm accepted sight unseen.

Just when I think it's all set, nature throws us what's now called a game-changer.

***

Dad and Barbara plan to move to a house in Stamford, Connecticut, where there will be room for the new baby. There is great excitement in the air. Barbara is pregnant! The house is being built! It's an opportunity I don't want to let pass. I've always wanted to live in a house instead of an apartment. Besides, New York City in the mid '70s is depressing, dangerous. What's more, Mom's not as fun as Dad and Barbara, not as upbeat and adventurous. She's been struggling to find a job and a man she can stand. Only I put it in better words when I finally muster the courage to tell her I want to move out and live with them.

"Are you sure?" Mom asks. Then: "Have I been so—? No. Never mind. Um, won't you miss Alec?"

I haven't thought of that. Alec? No, I guess not.

Yet having spoken my fantasy I'm suddenly not so sure about it. Dad is able to do more with me than Mom, better at tending to my physical requirements. That much is true. Yet Mom is more emotionally supportive. Even now, she suggests I see a psychologist to discuss this. Reluctantly, I agree. She has in mind a specialist named Dr. Friend. (I kid you not.)

***

"You'd be crazy to move now!" declares Dr. Friend several weeks later, after I speak my piece. A genial fellow with tufts of silver hair framing ample ears, he sits in a big black leather armchair by the window of his elegantly furnished suite off the lobby of an apartment building on Central Park West, a few blocks from home. Mom and Dad both promised he wouldn't tell me what to do, just help me make up my mind.

"Is—is that what you think?"

"Look, you're starting high school, which is big. Life is best taken a step at a time. Don't overwhelm yourself, particularly considering your upcoming surgery."

I don't want to think about *that*.

My scoliosis has become worse to the point of dangerous. The miserable back brace isn't working. I can put off an operation only so long.

When my attendant picks me up at Dr. Friend's office and pushes me home along CPW on what's turned into a blustery spring evening, almost immediately I decide to disobey the shrink.

≈≈≈ ● ≈≈≈

MY UNFORTUNATE, LIFE-CHANGING INCARCERATION

1976-1978

"Slow and steady wins the race."
—Aesop, "The Hare and the Tortoise"

My first day at Steiner, no one is expecting me. Housed in a converted townhouse on East 78th Street between Fifth and Madison avenues, the school is like a disheveled Old World dowager. It's warm and nurturing yet smells of mothballs.

I'm the first and only wheelchair student ever—pioneering, again!—and nobody's checked if the elevator is working. It's very old and arthritic, we're told. Like at Walden, Dad has to jerk my chair up the front steps, but we're used to that. Beggars can't be choosers. Inside is another story. We hadn't reckoned on an elevator problem.

The tiny "car"—a cargo elevator, if ever there was one—refuses to move from whatever floor it's on. When someone at last finds it and manages to open the tarnished old gate, my chair doesn't fit inside. I'm about ready to give up, whatever that means, when Dad removes my footrests and finagles till my chair and I are wedged in. That said, there is no extra space for another person to push the buttons, which I can't do myself. So long-legged Dad vaults the staircase to summon the elevator to the third floor. Still the rust bucket won't budge, until—honest to God—someone kicks the door from the outside!

Needless to say, I'm now late for my first class.

All of which gives me plenty of time to size up the people I'm hurriedly introduced to. So far, all the men wear the drab, narrow-lapelled suits of a previous generation; the two women in evidence are in navy pencil skirts and prim cream-color blouses that've seen better days as well. An odd sort of shabbiness, considering the affluent location, pervades. And not the hippy-dippy grunginess I'm used to from Walden.

My homeroom teacher—young, blondish, in a blousy neutral-toned dress shirt, conservative polka-dot tie, and comfortable shoes—interrupts his presentation to the class when I'm at last wheeled in. "Yes? Hi! Mattlin? Are you in the right class? Ninth grade? It's just that we weren't expecting you . . ."

No shit? I smile and remain silent. The other kids—roughly fifteen in all, I estimate—are staring at me from behind identical front-facing desks. (I'm relieved to notice no ties or blazers—a dress code somewhere between Walden's "anything going" and Alec's school's "young executives in training.") Most are girls, actually.

Much whispering ensues between the teacher and the swarm of 1950s-style administrators and others who've gathered. The source of the confusion is apparent, to me at least. I am the cause. I'm not supposed to be here. I'm supposed to be in Stamford.

Yesterday, I awoke to the darkness of 5:30 AM in Dad and pregnant Barbara's West End Avenue apartment (they'd moved from Brooklyn several years before), got in Dad's minibus-sized overcooked-broccoli-green Checker Marathon—the roomy "Limousine" edition, which could hold my wheelchair intact, without folding or removing the foot rests, if I ducked my head (and which Barbara, an opera buff, had dubbed *Brunhilda*)—and did the long reverse-commute to Connecticut. The house they're having built in Stamford isn't finished yet, and I didn't want to miss the first day of high school there. Rippowam High turned out to be a sprawling suburban campus of about a thousand students, quadruple the population of Walden's high school and about fourteen times Steiner's, spread out on a single floor. It's a public school, but it's supposed to be a good one. It's also pretty accessible. I'd roamed class to class in my motorized wheelchair, something I've never done before. But I got lost and my chair is slow, so I struggled to keep up. Many of the other kids already knew one another . . . and they'd looked different from kids I've known. What's more, outside the windows was nothing but trees and grass. You could hear birds, not car horns and sirens. So alien to me!

When my latest attendant, Kenny, brought me home to Manhattan's Upper West Side that afternoon, I was despondent. "How many trees can you stand?" I shrieked.

The realization: I am a city boy.

But I had a second chance at reinventing myself and finding happiness. Rudolf Steiner started one day later than Rippie. Why not give it a try, too? My parents agreed. What I hadn't realized is they never actually told Steiner about this second change of plans. They didn't have time.

At Steiner, the brouhaha soon settles down and I'm parked behind a desk at the end of the front row. Dad leaves. I struggle to learn the name of the girl on my right. She's pretty, and I figure if we're going to be neighbors we might as well be friends. The new me is as shy as the old me, however. The new me is still a work in progress.

The teacher re-begins his remarks. He's a broad-shouldered, slightly potbellied man, and his fair locks hang diagonally in a . . . well, a Hitleresque slant toward his bushy eyebrows. I've missed the part where he gives his name.

At lunch the other kids make a special effort to welcome me. "So what're your hobbies?" I'm asked probably six times. I become self-conscious about their solicitousness, but seize the opportunity. "Our teacher—what's his name?"

My question elicits giggles. A girl with flaming red hair and an expansive smile says, "Isn't it funny? German, I guess."

I wait. Then, in a hesitant, enchantingly soft voice, she says, "A Hard Penis." At least that's what I think she says. I nod knowingly, or try to as best I can, betraying no embarrassment. My head doesn't actually move much, so I sort of raise and lower my eyebrows, playing it cool. I'm good at using facial expressions to my advantage.

On the third day I have a pressing question about a homework assignment. I can't raise my hand. I raise a finger, but will have to call out. Maybe I can get by simply saying "Sir." No. Too formal. I decide to be brave. Perhaps if I say it fast enough, emphasizing the initial syllable and slurring the rest, I can get by. I'm good at fooling people. "Uh, Mr. PEEEN-ih—?"

He looks over. No one chortles. Maybe his name really *is* Mr. Penis.

There are a lot of funny names here. Kids called Almira and Bethea . . . at least I think I have those right. I hurriedly ask when book reports are due, and we go on to a lesson in recitation. Recitation is big here. Every morning starts not with the Pledge of Allegiance but with Steiner's own Morning Verse, which I soon learn. "I look into the world, in which the sun is shining, in which stars are sparkling, where stones repose . . ." The class speaks it in unison while standing up—slowly, reverentially, like some secret, ancient chant.

English class begins with a passage we're supposed to recite: "Respect for the word is the first commandment in the discipline by which a man can be educated to maturity—intellectual, emotional, and moral. Respect for the word—to employ it with scrupulous care and an incorruptible heartfelt love of truth—is essential if there is to be any growth in a society or in the human race . . ."

I sort of like that one. I've always had respect for scrupulously employed words! I become engaged in the lesson, and soon realize this oddly named teacher and eccentric, quasi-cultish school are growing on me. I made the right choice, coming here, staying in New York. I never think about moving to Stamford again.

Mr. Penis writes the name "Dag Hammarskjold" on the board. I only know it from the plaza near the UN. Someone then asks him to spell out his own name on the chalkboard. Thank God! Why couldn't I have done that?

He writes: EKKEHARD PIENING.

***

It's the autumn of 1976. Jimmy Carter is running for president against Gerald Ford. I'm convinced Carter will lose, because who would vote for a Southerner with blow-dried hair? "Shake Your Booty" by KC and the Sunshine Band is the top hit. I'm trying to be into what's happening now, and swear off talking about *Star Trek* as if it's real, though some of the popular disco music leaves me cold. I won't pretend I'm Chief Ironside or even the much cooler Steve McGarrett anymore. I spent last year signing "Steve" to my homework papers at Walden.

On the other hand, I don't want to be just Wheelchair Guy either. I like having a counter identity. If I can do something else—such as make my new classmates laugh—perhaps I can go from Wheelchair Guy to *Funny* Wheelchair Guy and, in time, to just plain Funny Guy.

I start doodling cartoons between classes and sometimes during classes. A few weeks later, the student paper publishes one. It's a caricature of Carter, Ford, and—what the hell—Nixon at a fictional debate. Nixon says, "I am not a crook." Ford says, "New York, drop dead." And Carter says, "Anybody want a peanut?"

I'm doing my best, but I'm fighting impossible odds. I'm still fat and wearing an uncomfortable back brace that makes my clothes fit funny. I take to holding my bathroom needs till I get home, on the assumption I'm too old to ask teachers for that kind of help. On occasion I have accidents, concocting clever excuses and misdirection. "I spilled my drink!" Or "What's that smell? Did my chair run through dog doo in the park?"

Soon medical imperative blows my cover.

***

My curving spine has overpowered the pinching back brace. My weak muscles can't keep up. My back has nearly folded over itself. I look more like a beach ball than an almost-fifteen-year-old boy. And the orthopedist says the situation has become critical. Without surgery, and soon, breathing will become increasingly problematic as my body closes in against my lungs. I'll become unable to sit in a chair within five years. My parents have insisted on getting second opinions. Now three of New York's top orthopedic surgeons agree.

We pick Dr. David Levine of the Hospital for Special Surgery. He seems the most responsive to questions, even from me, and I like his sunny manner. His penchant for bowties is either a plus or a minus—I can't decide.

To prepare for next summer's surgery, I spend the better part of spring break in the hospital for tests. I'm given a private room in the pediatric ward. Disney characters are painted on the walls. Come on, I'm nearly fifteen!

Out my window you can see the East River. The hospital is on prime real estate! Mostly I like the small Sony Trinitron color TV on a pivoting gooseneck over the adjustable bed. I can't change channels myself, but at least I can pick what and when to watch and ask a nurse for help.

For five days I undergo a litany of tests—breathing tests, blood tests, and so forth. I try to find the bright side, look at the nurses as sex objects, because that's what the cool guys at school would do, but I'm too busy taking it all in and being bored to float any pleasure.

While I'm there, Mom checks into New York Hospital, which is adjacent. She says she can see my room out her window, but I don't see hers.

She has a tumor removed from her ovaries. She's forty-three, scared because ovarian cancer is what killed her mother. I'm convinced she's worrying over nothing. She usually does. Mom calls her operation a "procedure." What we don't know is it'll be the first in a long series of procedures. One afternoon, accompanied by a nurse, Mom drags her IV over the bridge connecting the two buildings and visits me in pediatrics. She's weak and pale but tries to be cheerful, and I do too.

We're also unaware that, that same April, disability activists are protesting at federal office buildings in ten major cities. The Rehabilitation Act of 1973 still has not been signed into law, four years after Congress passed it. Specifically, the guidelines necessary to enforce Section 504 of the Act, which bars discrimination against people with disabilities in federally funded programs, haven't been finalized. Without those guidelines, the nation's first disability-rights legislation is rendered meaningless.

Protesters believe newly installed President Carter may be sympathetic to their cause, but so far he's done nothing.

The San Francisco demonstrations are the largest. Scores of activists occupy the local headquarters of the US Department of Health, Education, and Welfare, the body responsible for the guidelines. They camp out for twenty-five straight days and nights, sleeping in their wheelchairs or on the floor. They share urinals, catheters, and personal-care attendants, bathing in front of each other without shame—most are used to being undressed in front of others. I know the feeling.

These activists are inspired by the Black civil-rights movement, of course, but more than that, they have nothing to lose and nothing else to do. They're unemployed or, in many cases, barred from all but a handful of mainstream schools. Having benefited from the latest medical advances, they've survived crippling, once deadly diseases and accidents to live active lives with the aid of crutches, power wheelchairs, portable ventilators, guide dogs, sign language, and other modern marvels. Many don't have their own homes or families to tend to. They feel they've been patient long enough.

At the end of the month the protesters are victorious! Joseph Califano, Carter's HEW secretary, finalizes the regulations and the president signs them into law. A modicum of rights, at last! Power to the people! It will prove only the first battle of a long war, of an ongoing revolution, but it's one from which I'll personally benefit very soon. For all institutions that receive federal funds are now required to become handicapped accessible by 1980. That's the year I start college.

***

Meanwhile, in the months that follow, I feel I'm making a little history myself—or at least approaching a Big Event. The hospital days in April were just preliminary. The Big Event is this summer's surgery.

No one has ever spent a summer in a hospital like I'm going to spend the summer in the hospital. There will be a series of operations culminating in a spinal fusion—which will attach pieces of metal called Harrington rods to my pretzel-like spine. The rods won't make me completely straight but significantly straight*er*, which is the best we can hope for. I'll be in the hospital for three or four months, with a two-month interval at a rehabilitation facility. In all, six months under institutional medical care. Summer *and* fall. Or so goes the plan.

It's enough to make an ordinary teenager crumble, perhaps, but not me. This is my big battle, the travail I must endure to achieve stature, literally. I'm Ben-Hur facing the Roman galley ship. If he can row for three years, I can lie in an institutional bed for six months. In characteristic fashion, macho fantasies come to my rescue.

At Mom's urging, I start scribbling my fears and expectations in a notebook. I will keep a journal before, during, and after. At the very least it gives me something to do with my pent-up energies, at once a focus and a distraction.

I begin wondering what I might actually lose from gaining a straighter back, and experiment in the bathtub with auto-fellatio. Contact! A dirty little secret of the extremely scoliotic! Yet I come away without a clear understanding of what all the fuss is about blow jobs.

When school's out, in early-June, I have a couple of weeks free and arrange to see *Star Wars* with a girl from school, my first half-assed attempt at a date. We get our signals crossed, however, and I become impatient waiting for her to call back. I end up seeing it alone and don't enjoy it. My pre-hospital time feels too precious to waste on waiting around for the phone to ring.

Finally, I am again admitted to a private room in pediatrics. For the first few days, more tedious tests—X-rays, blood panels, whatever. Every time I pee it's measured, and when I don't a nurse asks me if I want to. They expect you to piss every hour! Then I get a preview of my coming traction, so to speak—a system to stretch my spine mechanically over the course of a week before the rods are actually inserted. It sounds laughably primitive, but Dr. Levine insists it's necessary and he's done it hundreds of times. Or I should say, he's done it to hundreds of other patients. He even produces a past patient as a sort of reference, I suppose, and to cheer me up and reassure me that this is not the end of the world.

I'm awake when Levine drills holes into my skull—the first step of traction. I've been injected with a local anesthetic, and I feel nothing. Then a heavy metal ring is installed on my head—actually screwed into my cranium. They call it a halo. But aren't halos supposed to be light as air, luminous, and ethereal? This is about as light as an iron.

A matching set of metal pins is installed near my knees. Again, "pins" is a misnomer. Pins are small and narrow. These are not. These hurt like hell. They are metal dowels that, like the halo, go through the bone; they stick out on either side. I complain for days about my right knee in particular. It throbs so much Dr. Levine decides to redo that portion. He moves the pin a centimeter or two. It's still sensitive to the touch but less painful most of the time.

Cords are tied onto the halo and leg pins, attached to pulleys with a weight at the other end. Yes, I'm being drawn and quartered! I'm lying on my back all the time now. My upper body may be elevated slightly, but the idea is to keep my spine stretched as straight as possible so it'll be amenable to the Harrington rods, which will be surgically implanted a couple of weeks later. In this position, it's impossible to keep my journal. I'm again glad for the Sony Trinitron. I think I learn every episode of the *Mary Tyler Moore Show* by heart.

I try dictating to a small tape recorder, but it's not the same. I listen to music cassettes through an earphone, mostly Beatles. Which is not in keeping with the zeitgeist, of course, but since I was too young to fully appreciate the Beatles in their time it's not exactly nostalgia either. Besides, sometimes the coolest thing to do is not follow what everybody else is doing. I'm beginning to learn that.

In any case, no one from school will know.

When Mom and Dad visit—usually on alternate days—they bring me more Beatles cassettes and other music I request, such as Aerosmith, which I'm just starting to get into. Alec is in England and France with a high-school tour group. He promises to bring back British versions of Beatles LPs.

The day of the big surgery, Mom and Dad appear together very early in the morning, for pre-op. I'm sedated. It doesn't make me sleepy. It makes me giddy. As I'm being rolled off toward the operating room, I tell my parents, "I have one question. Before he cuts me open, I need to know if he's a *kosher* butcher!"

They find this hysterically funny. Dad laughs like a seal. He pats my foot, which is under several layers of sheets. He's always patting me. Mom shakes her head and says how very funny I am. Grace under pressure, she says. Not really. It's more a burnished reflex. Make light of a difficult situation. Find the humorous side of it. Put people at ease.

The lights in the OR are very bright. I want sunglasses. Instead, I meet the anesthesiologist. A face behind a surgical mask. He asks me to count backward from one-hundred. I get to ninety-six.

When I wake up, I'm being lifted by a gang of a half-dozen or more in surgical outfits. Lifted from one bed to another. There's a pain in my lower back, near my waist. I try to say "My waist! My waist!" but no words come out. I have a tracheostomy. Dr. Levine had explained this. I was likely to come out of surgery with a buildup of fluids in my lungs, and since I'm unable to cough, a tracheostomy will allow the doctors to suction out the gunk from my lungs. So for now I cannot speak.

Dr. Levine sees that I'm trying to talk. He tells the others to stop. He leans over me, and I can make out his rosy-cheeked face, his red curly hair, his clownish bow tie. I don't have my glasses on, but these things are unmistakable. "What is it? What're you trying to say?"

I like Dr. Levine for trying to understand. Yet I'm too dazed to think up an alternate explanation, a suitable vocabulary. I keep mouthing *My waist, my waist*. Finally he gets it. He feels under me, around my waist, but finds nothing wrong. "See if it gets better. It should go away." (It does, but I don't notice when.)

The next twelve hours are the most horrifying. The Recovery Room. A tube is inserted in my nose. Maybe it's been there all day but I'm just now feeling it. It makes it hard to swallow my own saliva. The room is dark and crowded. Lots of people on lots of beds, countless machines beeping and humming. No

TVs. I float in and out of sleep. Well, of consciousness. I'm not permitted to see my parents until morning. I'm not sure I'll make it till morning.

I hear someone in another bed—an old woman, it sounds like—discussing the difference between "mottled" and "modeled." She's trying to explain a mark or a feeling on her skin and the nurse isn't getting it. I want to help. I'm good at explaining. Mom always says words are my strongest tool, and I have learned time and again it is so. *Respect for the word* . . . But I can't help this poor woman across the Recovery Room. I can't get up and I can't speak. This must be what it feels like to be buried alive, I think.

I try to memorize everything that's going on around me, so I can put it in words later, in my notebook, but without my glasses I can't see and without my brain fully switched on I have a hard time stringing together pairs of sentences in my head. Forget paragraphs. *Later*, I think. *I will write all this later.* But first I have to stop feeling like I've been run over by a Mack truck. Whatever a Mack truck is exactly . . .

Mack the Knife. Maybe that's better. Stabbed by Mack the Knife.

When morning comes, I'm thrilled to see light. Whether it's the fluorescent bulbs outside the Recovery Room or the summer sun shining through the windows, I can't be certain. Either way it's bright and new and I'm rolled out of the Recovery Room and I'm okay. Mom and Dad are there—here, coming up to my rolling bed. I'm transferred to another bed, one in the ICU, which is a big room with five or six patients near the nurse's station. Each bed has its own little Sony Trinitron color TV. Feels almost like being home again.

Dr. Levine visits. He says he was able to do the two parts of the spinal fusion at once, in that one surgery. We're ahead of schedule. "But your bones are like eggshells," he cautions. "You need more milk."

Later I'm given a small plastic plug to close off the trach so I can talk. It doesn't come to me right away, and I struggle and gasp until at last I can speak in small increments.

Whenever I feel pain, which isn't often, I'm given a dose of Demerol in my IV. It's the most wonderful sensation I've ever experienced—a luscious, tingly warmth that spreads within until I fall blissfully asleep. Soon I have to cut back on the doses; requests for more receive a "can you wait a bit longer?" or outright denial. That's okay. I'm comfortable.

After a week I'm still on an IV and a large, noisy ventilator, which I hadn't noticed before. Tubes everywhere. Machines beeping and buzzing . . . It's amazing I can sleep at all, and on my back yet! They're not all my machines, I gradually perceive. Some belong to my neighbors in the ICU. We don't interact. Maybe the families do, but not me. Mom and Dad might say a word to my roommates' visitors, but I'm in my own world.

One night the lights go off and on again. Nurses are suddenly swarming all around me. The head nurse is called in, though she's supposed to be off-duty. It's a blackout, they say. Indeed, the nursing staff is jabbering about it. I vaguely remember the blackout of '65. I was not yet three. It seemed Dad would never come home from the office. But he did and all was well.

So I'm not worried now. But my nurses are. Very. They pump a sort of football-shaped manual respirator into my trach. They check my pulse repeatedly. They check blood gases, which involves a painful needle into the muscles of my groin. They're relieved to discover my oxygen level is fine. The hospital has its own power generator, and soon my respirator is on again. It breathes for me and I become lazy. But I insist I'm fine. I'm not lightheaded. I'm not short of breath. At least I think I'm insisting. Mostly I'm smiling.

Soon the ventilator is removed completely, and I breathe on my own. I'm fine. Yes, fine. Always fine. At times I'm even allowed to roll onto my belly, propped on a special wedge-shaped pillow. As long as my spine is kept in alignment, it's okay. With the pillow wedge, I can place my notebook down on the mattress and do a little writing.

One of my biggest concerns remains: Can I still touch my dick now that my back's straightened? (With my hand, that is, not my mouth—"reach myself," as Dad might put it.) Eureka! I can! I can! When the nurses remove the surgical catheter and wrap a soft, loose cloth diaper around my crotch, it enhances the experience!

***

After two months at Special Surgery, I'm transferred to a convalescent facility in Westchester County. I've been so cloistered, the glimpses of New York in August passing through the ambulance windows blow my mind. The city looks beautiful . . . absolutely mesmerizing and inspiring. I feel like a tourist in my own town!

A tourist who's strapped to a gurney, that is.

Sadly, the euphoria is temporary. Soon we're in the suburbs. By and by we arrive at Happyvale, the institution I'll call home for the next three months. The very name conjures a shadow-gray sanitarium from an old horror movie. I'm rolled inside and eventually parked in a large room with pale-blue walls and seven other kids. It's a downgrade from the ICU. Only one TV, for starters.

One of my new roommates, a young boy in pressed blue jeans and a tucked-in button shirt with yellow stripes, greets Dad, who is accompanying me on the trip, with a stagy formal bow. "Hello, my good man!" the boy says. This kid is so animated and *not* post-op-like and, well, on his feet . . . the nettling question for me is, why am I in the same place he is?

It's soon apparent that the staff here is less well trained than the hospital crew I've grown used to; they're rougher, sloppier. My trach is never cleaned. I'm not bathed as thoroughly, if at all. And the place doesn't have wedge pillows (unless, I later learn, you place a special order). Plus it's harder for my parents to visit, being out in the suburbs. Within two days I'm begging for a transfer.

Can't I stay in the city? Or perhaps be cared for at home? Dad calls Dr. Levine. My request is denied. There's no extra room at any city hospitals. I need to stay here, to recover slowly and be professionally monitored. I'll have to make the best of it. I imagine I've been captured by the Gamesters of Triskelion . . . Oops—I forgot. No *Star Trek*.

Happyvale has a sort of school I'm rolled to every day in my hospital bed, even though it's summer. One thing I like about it is it has an extensive tape library. Through headphones, I listen to articles about politics, science, technology. Soon I have a volunteer—a groovy dude dressed in denim, with big dark glasses and a shaggy haircut, who smells of cigarettes, which is a scent I like, and calls me "buddy"—to read to me from *The Pickwick Papers*, my assigned summer reading (it's not in the audio library).

When Mom visits, she brings food—kosher London broil and baked chicken, personal favorites, which aren't on the establishment's menu. I keep a stash of Doritos by my bedside, which, believe it or not, *is* marked kosher. I need someone to feed me, since I'm lying down. I learn it's easier to swallow when rolled on one side.

I have to be rolled like a log, because the metal halo is now attached to a plaster cast that covers my torso and part of one leg. The leg pins have been removed, but my neck and, to a degree, hips are immobilized.

At one point I'm made to visit the institution's psychologist. I'm wheeled in my hospital bed to his large, quiet office. He's a surprisingly nice, young guy—bushy curly hair and beard of a color somewhere between brown and black. The facial hair does not obscure his eager smile. "Do you play chess?" he asks.

Rolled onto my side, propped up on pillows, I can see the chessboard well enough to tell him my moves. It's a good game and it gets me out of my usual schedule of inane classes. I suspect it gets him out of his usual schedule, too. He seems to enjoy my company. (I'm embarrassed that now I can't remember his name, or who won the game. Perhaps we played two.)

On a later visit he administers a rudimentary IQ test. After, he tells me I'm well above average. I don't believe him. I think he's just being nice. If anybody looked like he needed someone to be nice to him, it was I. He says no, he's not just being nice. He insists his test doesn't lie. And I begin to think maybe everyone else isn't as smart as I assume they are.

***

Because of being so stationary, I take physical therapy three times a week. Which reminds me of the pointless exercises of my early childhood, except this time I'm at an age to enjoy the attentions of my therapist, a really attractive brunette. As she flexes my knees and elbows, and orders me to work my fingers by buttoning and unbuttoning a raggedy old shirt, I only grumble slightly and, I hope, with the utmost charm.

The solitary television set in my room, mounted high, is on pretty much all the time. It's the summer of the Son of Sam killer. Elvis Presley dies. A new actress will replace Farrah on *Charlie's Angels*, and I enjoy reading in *People* magazine about her measurements (Cheryl Ladd's bust is even bigger than Farrah's!). But the weight of all this, the impact, is the dour realization that the world outside these institutional walls goes on, while I go nowhere.

One of my cellmates, er, roommates, with whom I have a begrudging affinity because he likes the Beatles and covets my tape collection, wonders aloud about the meaning of Elvis' demise. "Does it mean Elton John is now the king of pop? They always called him the prince, so—"

Try as I might, I can't block out all of it. One sound in particular will haunt me for years to come. It involves poor Murph, another of my roommates, a young man who is rumored to have lived at Happyvale *most of his seventeen years*! It's said he *could* go home but his family doesn't want him . . . it's said they visit only on Christmas, Easter, and maybe his birthday. I don't know if any of this is true, but he never leaves his bed for a wheelchair (then again, neither do I), and his infrequent speech is hopelessly garbled, probably from cerebral palsy or a brain injury. You don't need to understand his words to hear the urgency, anger, frustration, sorrow.

Yet worst of all is how the nurses tease him, loudly, every few days when they discover wet semen on his sheets, his catheter blocked or popped off. "Hee-ha!" the loudest one laughs. "What you been doin'?! You gotta cut that out! I ain't cleanin' up this mess no mo'! You a bad boy!"

(That's how I remember hearing it anyway, a dialect I normally find comfortingly authentic and down-home suddenly turned sharp and menacing.)

I vow never again to be jealous of the cool, popular boys at school or resent others' mobility and freedom. I've come to realize that I could have a lot less mobility and freedom than I do. I will remember how lucky I am. I'll put the inimical, tough-guy Ben to rest forever when I return to the land of the living, and always try to appreciate my life just as it is. As long as it's far away from here or any place like it.

I make this vow privately and never tell anyone. But it's dead serious. The most religious experience I think I'll ever have. A promise I make to God. "Let me out of here, and I'll never forget."

On Labor Day weekend, Barbara and Dad visit with their new baby, Jeff. Barbara barbecues a chicken in Happyvale's outdoor area. My bed is rolled outside, too. We all try to pretend it's pleasant and normal.

***

Life, however compromised, settles into a pattern.

Back in New York, the school year is starting without me. One afternoon in early-September, Mom brings a manila envelope stuffed with my classmates' good wishes. I know it was an assignment from Mr. Penis, but I'm moved nevertheless and reread every note. I call it my fan mail, and still have the package today.

In response, lying there like a slab, I ask Mom to take dictation. I want to write a sort of thank-you to my class, or really an explanation of what I've been going through—to head off rumors, excess sympathy, and most of all awkward silences upon my return. I want to submit it to the school newspaper. Still figuring humor is the key to improving my social standing, I give it the sarcastic title "What I Did Over My Summer Vacation," and begin it with, "Have you ever wondered how dirt gets on the ceiling?"—a reference to the boredom of lying supine day after day. I end with, "Try not to be too jealous."

Toward the end of my stay, I gather sufficient courage to ask one of the volunteer teaching aides if she'd like to go to a movie "when I'm back on the outside." She's a pretty, dark-haired high-school girl with a warm smile, and says yeah, sure, but I'm not confident she means it and I wonder how I'd follow through anyway since she lives in Westchester. Still, it's good practice, I figure, since I didn't do so well with my *Star Wars* date.

***

When at last I'm returned to Special Surgery, I'm put in a regular room in pediatrics with one other boy and no individual Trinitron, just one big set for the room. One evening he asks me what it's like to be a teenager. He must be about twelve. I don't know what to answer. *Me, a teenager?* It's then I realize my lengthy incarceration has made me older in some indefinable way, or at least *feel* older.

The halo and trach are removed and the cast cut back, though I must continue wearing what's left, which is most of it, for several more months. Still, the end of my hospitalization is near! After four months that were supposed to have been six.

I'm truly lucky.

You see, the odd assortment of suffering I witnessed, especially at Happyvale, will leave an indelible mark. I'll never forget Murph, my masturbating Happyvale roommate. After sharing a slice of life with kids like that, I cannot be the same again. I know exactly how the other half lives, and it's not good. For those of us with severe disabilities, you can never be too safe, too well protected, because the institutional snuffing out of privacy and dignity can never feel so very far away.

I've lost a lot of weight, too, despite the Doritos—which feels good, since I was fat—and I'm taller than I was, since my back is straighter. I also now sport several long, downy tufts on my chin and will need to shave as soon as I'm released. A new man, within spitting distance of fifteen.

***

When I return to high school, it's late-October. The weather has turned chilly and gray. The kids are already settled into a new routine, but there's little change from last year. It's the same teacher, Ekkehard Piening; the same kids—there is only one class per grade—and, at Steiner, the routine scarcely varies from year to year or, I suspect, generation to generation.

To my surprise, I'm greeted by an abundance of bonhomie. The essay I dictated to Mom about my hospital experience has appeared in the school paper, and my words worked their magic!

I have to wear the upper-body cast, which protrudes from my shirt, but I have no shame about it and the kids are accepting. At recess I have someone tip my wheelchair back against the wall to ease the pressure on my spine—doctor's orders—and even that goes smoothly. Plus my terrific attendant, Kenny, decides to stay on, despite the four-month hiatus. He doesn't stay with me at school but takes me there and back every day and works late when Mom goes out at night. A medical student on leave, he's smart and we talk about everything. He becomes the *nice* big brother I never had. I begin to see how important the quality of my attendant is to my very quality of life.

Every second weekend I visit Stamford, where Dad's my attendant. Jeff is growing up, which is fun to see, but I have no friends and nothing to do there and it's boring. My friends have become very important to me.

With each year of high school my roster of friends increases. More and more, I let them push my wheelchair in Central Park or on the street, which gives me a feeling of autonomy from the parental security blanket. I get a little nervous when they're pushing my chair over the potholes and bumps, but I never let on.

At school, one of my friends, Nanci, remembers my penchant for cartooning and wants a drawing of a shirtless Robert Plant, based on a magazine picture she cherishes. Flattered, I take special care on the important details, which doesn't go unnoticed. She squeals in delight when I present her with my penciled masterpiece. "Look—he even got the bulge in his jeans!"

Alec, still the big brain, aces his SAT and will probably go to Harvard, like Dad. I don't want to go that route or be like that. I've learned to stop being a dork, trying to impress others with my intellectual chops, which I'm not sure I have anyway. The new Ben goes with the flow, lets the good times roll, and never forgets that misery and suffering are as close as my shadow.

When time comes for me to take the SAT, Mother—as I've taken to calling her, to show my maturity—gets me tutored. She knows I haven't had Alec's academic training. Mom has become happier, except for the weekends of chemo- and radiation-induced nausea, during which she hides in her bedroom. She's become an item with a man named Bob, another writer and Harvard grad. She's also working full-time at a small publishing house. Though she complains that it doesn't pay much, she insists she enjoys the camaraderie and intellectual stimulation. She's even trying to write her own book about having cancer. She says when it's published she'll take us to Europe.

For her, seeing me grow up and managing a degree of independence is a relief and a joy, she says. As if she doesn't want to leave this world worrying about me.

I tell her the first time I smoke cigarettes with friends in the Park. I know she won't get mad, and in fact I'm almost showing off, like smoking with the guys is a badge of the acceptance I've achieved. Sure enough, she likes it; she's glad I have enough autonomy to be a little naughty. Fitting in and being well socialized have always been important to her.

It's very nice that Mother and I now have this kind of understanding and honesty between us. I'm glad I didn't "divorce" her and move to Stamford. Dr. Friend, the shrink, knew what he was talking about!

When I at last take the SAT, Mother makes sure a proctor goes over my answer bubbles. I'm able to handle a regular pencil (or lightweight pen) and paper pretty well, but she's worries I don't press hard enough to make my answers register.

Soon all such standardized tests will be required to make accommodations like that for students like me. But at the time, we have to take accommodations into our own hands.

≈≈≈ • ≈≈≈

THE END OF CHILDHOOD

1979-1980

"I'm not what you'd call a brilliant thinker—such results as I get are usually the fruits of patience, industry, and unimaginative plugging, helped out now and then, maybe, by a little luck—but I do have my flashes of intelligence."
—Dashiell Hammett,
"Zigzags of Treachery," *Detective Stories*

"If you apply here," the heavyset man in a boxy charcoal-gray suit is telling me between slow, heaving breaths, "you'll get in."

Dappled sun seeps through the cream-colored curtains behind him. It's early morning. Still. Barely a heartbeat has passed since I was wheeled into this musty office—Dean What's-His-Name's words catch me off-guard. I look to his semi-serious, muffin expression for a clue as to how to react. Was it a prediction, a joke, or a promise? My eyes dart away, down at my still fingers folded haphazardly in my blue-jeaned lap. Semi-casual in my attire: sport coat, good shirt, good jeans. Exuding self-confidence. Iconoclastic. I imagine my listless hands gesturing dramatically. Pointing. Clapping.

Did he actually say . . . ? Warm excitement rises within me.

"Oh?"

"Yes. You hear me? How's that make you feel? About what I said. Surprised?"

Again, I'm speechless. The thing is, I haven't had a chance to utter Word One of my carefully crafted, privately rehearsed spiel! I haven't told him how great I am, or why I want to go to Amherst (not that I'm absolutely certain I do) . . . what I'd bring to the place! I haven't unleashed any of my knock-his-socks-off questions!

I'm a little cloudy-headed. Last night, after five hours' drive in a blinding downpour, with Kenny at the wheel of the old, unreliable, Checker behemoth, we'd spent the night at a motel. Just Kenny and I. It's the first time I've traveled so far from home without parents, and I'm still proud-excited-scared.

Mother had said I was responsible for finding the motel and getting to my appointment on time. She wasn't sure Kenny had ever checked into a motel before! As if people from Trinidad, by way of Brooklyn, don't know the ways of the world. *It's your responsibility. You have to be alert and speak up.* Just like with my seat belt all those years ago

Once checked in, though it was nearly ten PM, I dutifully phoned home to announce I was still alive, then watched an hour of crappy TV—the sort I knew Mother wouldn't approve of, not that there was much TV she *did* like—and slept with the contentment of one who knows he's done a good job. Kenny was in the next bed, ready to respond if I called out to roll over. But I didn't.

In the morning, directing Kenny to dress me to casual perfection, I knew I'd never have had a chance at this kind of freedom if Dad had come along, as originally planned. In this wonderful (assisted) self-determination, this semi-autonomy, I saw my adult future, and I liked it.

And now, here in Amherst's rarefied admissions office, I'm tongue-tied. "I assume"—I venture—"I assume I'd be the only handicapped student here?"

"Yes. Quite frankly, we don't have a lot of experience with people like you, people with your particular affliction."

Not crazy about the word "affliction," but I soldier on. "I'm used to being a kind of pioneer."

Zing! It's one of my rehearsed taglines, and I more-or-less led him to it! No pitiful handicapped-afflicted boy, me; I'm a *pioneer*, boldly going where no man has gone before!

I tentatively release my remaining arsenal, climaxing with the four killer questions guaranteed to get you accepted, according to a friend of Mother's— notwithstanding that my acceptance might no longer be in doubt.

"I've always gone to progressive schools"—my embellishment—"so I wonder, what is Amherst's *educational philosophy*?"

The Dean clasps his hands behind his close-cropped head and sighs audibly. "Good question," he says and then mutters something about education and individuality and maturation and citizenship, blah blah blah.

"Well," I follow up, "what would you say is the *political climate* at Amherst? Left, right, or center?"

He pauses, leans forward thoughtfully. "You mean among the administration, faculty, or students?"

My insides freeze. In my small high school, the faculty *is* the administration. "All of the above."

I have no idea what his answer is. I'm not listening, except for the next silence, which cues question number three

"Who really *runs* the college—the students, the faculty, or"—I add abruptly—"the administration? Who has the *power*?"

The Dean's answer comes slowly, whatever it is. Doesn't matter. I'm busy trying to remember the fourth question. Damn! Well, good enough.

Yet another question lingers long after I leave his office and Kenny drives me the long way home to Central Park West: Is Amherst honestly pre-accepting me simply because I'm handicapped?

***

What I don't know is, at about the same time, a disabled person named Davis is suing a school called Southeastern Community College for failure to provide equal access. The case goes before the US Supreme Court, which sides with the plaintiff and establishes a precedent for requiring "reasonable modifications."

Simultaneously, more or less, Congress establishes federal funding for independent-living programs, like the one in Berkeley, and creates the National Council of the Handicapped, which is charged with overseeing accessibility in public education.

Also in the late 1970s, the Disability Rights Education and Defense Fund is established, in Berkeley (where else?). It still leads the fight today.

Meanwhile, at Denver's Atlantis Community—an independent-living center modeled on Berkeley's—emboldened activists launch demonstrations against the local transit authority for failure to install wheelchair lifts on public buses. Guys and gals in wheelchairs actually sit in the middle of the street blocking buses! Their fire spreads to other cities and, by the early '80s, will spark a national grassroots organization called ADAPT, or American Disabled for Accessible Public Transit. A decade later, most city buses will have wheelchair lifts and wheelchair-lock-down apparatuses. To keep the momentum going, though, ADAPT will morph into a network dedicated to fighting the institutionalization of people with disabilities in favor of in-home long-term care. Now standing for American Disabled for Attendant Programs Today, ADAPT remains active.

And in 1978, my junior year of high school, Harper & Row publishes Professor Frank Bowe's *Handicapping America: Barriers to Disabled People.* Bowe, one of the leaders in the protests that led to implementation of Section 504 of the Rehab Act, is blind. His exploration of the policies and attitudes that deny people with disabilities full equality becomes a kind of *Souls of Black Folk* for the fledgling disability-rights movement. In 2007, when Bowe will die at age sixty, he'll be a tenured professor of disability studies at Hofstra University—an academic discipline that might not exist without his seminal work.

But at sixteen, I'm stupefyingly unaware and dismissive of these and most other sociopolitical events. I might have a vague sense that there are activists somewhere in the cosmos agitating for better treatment for people "like me," but what's that got to do with me personally? Besides, I have bigger things on my mind. Thinking about college has me as self-involved as a bride.

***

//You're kidding?" is Alec's reaction, on the phone from Harvard, to my news about Amherst. He would've been well suited to shtetl life, I think for the first of what will become dozens of times. Anything new, different, or unexpected is inconceivable and suspect.

Yet I'm suspicious too. Being in a wheelchair has always made good things happen. I've been hustled to the front of long movie lines, ushered through backstage doors to meet Broadway stars, and even given free toys and snacks. People feel sorry for me. I know I should say *No—don't treat me like a delicate child!* But I prefer to think of it as being a VIP.

Only Mother asks if I *want* to go to Amherst. I'm honestly not sure.

Dad's the one who got the ball rolling, making the first calls to the schools on my list. He asks, innocently enough, *if* they can take me—almost apologetic in his approach. Amherst's answer was to invite me for an interview. The rest feign a laissez-faire openness, many offering lawsuit-fearing bullshit reassurances. Except one: Duke University. "It'll be damn difficult," Dad quotes back to me. Needless to say, I don't apply there.

Dad claims he doesn't care where I go—then jokes, of Amherst, "even if it's one of Massachusetts' *lesser* institutions." In our family, humor covers a lot of unpleasantness.

I know Dad is a proud Harvard man. His time there, in the 1940s, was liberating and stimulating, after his anti-intellectual boyhood in Ohio. But I'm having a hard time seeing it that way.

Over the next few months, Kenny and I dutifully visit Harvard, Yale, and Princeton—practically the only colleges that exist on Dad's map. At Harvard we spend the night in a Lowell House suite occupied by friends of Alec's. It's up a few steps, but Alec's own room is up a couple of flights. I remember brushing my hair in the morning, with Kenny holding my arm to reach, and grimacing at my blow-dried mane's frizziness. A bad omen, it seems.

The gloomy day is filled with bad omens. I detest the bumpy cobblestone and brick pathways, which make my wheelchair feel like it has a flat tire. I also don't like eating at large group tables in the echoey dining halls. You see, the way I feed myself—hunched forward just so, my left hand supporting my right arm, with which I raise a lightweight fork or spoon to my mouth in slow steps, often walking my fingers up my chest—takes time and concentration. Plus I have to swallow carefully, to be sure nothing gets stuck in my throat or slides down to my lungs. This is one of the more delightful side effects of my spinal muscular atrophy!

As the weeks wear on, I develop an increasingly deep, sickening doubt about whether I can survive among these dreary colonial digs and seedy, tweedy Old World traditions. The expectation of becoming an Ivy League up-and-comer battles the frightening reality of my physical limitations and sense of vulnerability.

Which is why my mood is brightened when Mother inadvertently suggests a solution of sorts. "What about Stanford and Berkeley?"

Perhaps she was reading my mind, but contrary teenager that I am, I scoff. "Do you think I can't handle the Ivy League?"

"Not at all. The weather's better in California. *I'd* give them a look."

A few evenings later her "gentleman friend" Bob is over for dinner. He asks about my college choices, including the California schools, and weighs in with, "Avoid the snow." Are all adults hypocrites? I'm surrounded by them!

"I'm not going for a vacation," I say, insulted. *You think I can't handle snow?*

He absorbs my tone and takes a pensive swallow of his bourbon and water. "Springtime in Cambridge *is* lovely."

I tell him California seems far away, which actually was Dad's reaction. Bob pooh-poohs.

"It's only a five-hour flight versus a five-hour car or train ride."

Good point, I think. Still, isn't he missing something? What if something should happen to me three-thousand miles from my family?

***

A month later Dad takes me to California. He's set up a meeting with a Stanford graduate student who uses a wheelchair. The slight, balding man has a small apartment off campus. It has remote-controlled lights and doors. As if that weren't enough, he tells me the BART subway system is wheelchair accessible. I've pretty much lived my life assuming subways were off-limits unless I was with someone strong enough to hoist my chair up and down the stairs, so I'm intrigued as by a magic trick. Still, I'm self-conscious meeting this guy and fail to appreciate the research Dad has done.

Afterward, Dad wheels me around campus. It's bright and warm and looks like Fantasy Island. Plus the pavement is distinctly smooth and even. We loll by a fountain under a palm tree. There's a cart selling fresh oranges—I've grown up with hot-dog stands and Italian-ice carts, not fruit on the street!—and we share a juicy one in the luminous open air. When a sun-bleached coed strolls by, her silken light-brown hair bouncing off her tanned shoulders, we both grin stupidly and are surprised when she says hi to the obvious strangers.

"I think I'm in love," says Dad, after she's out of range. (I hope!)

For me, it's a memorable golden moment, seeing Dad let his hair down. Does it mark a shift in our relationship?

The good vibrations are short-lived. Soon we're loading back into the rented car—he folds my chair into the trunk, after lifting me into the shotgun seat. Despite complaining about feeling sweaty, Dad refuses to take off his blazer or even loosen his tie while driving. I tease him, play on our newfound familiarity by pointing out the incongruity. "I need to maintain my New Yorker identity," he explains.

And I wonder how much we're both pretending something.

***

Next, Dad takes me to the independent-living center in Berkeley. How he keeps coming up with these places is beyond me. Also, why? I am sixteen.

We meet a mountain of a woman in a motorized wheelchair. She's wearing a sort of tie-dyed tent dress—and mostly addresses *me*, not Dad. She asks if I know my rights.

I know them from my lefts. I memorized the difference because the hand control on my electric wheelchair at home is on my right side. It's important to know your left and right when you're giving other people instructions about which way to manipulate your body.

Naturally, I don't say any of this.

The woman looks beguilingly powerful in her wheeled throne. She's all about power Out of nowhere she tells me how important it is to ask for help when you need it—how it doesn't show powerlessness but actually gives you power. I'm not sure about that, but I have to admit I've always been shy about asking strangers to open doors for me, and such. Being "assertive," as she calls it, simultaneously raises other people's consciousness of access barriers and empowers you to go out in the world independently, to stop relying on family or hired assistants. I nod, in my subtle way. But this is sounding dangerously close to a condescending lecture, and I tune out, focus on her gadgets. I particularly like the speakerphone. (Just like Ironside's!) She notices, and demonstrates how it's activated with a simple switch even I could push.

I still don't know how I'll live on campus—*any* campus—without my family. Without Kenny. But perhaps I'm beginning to get a picture. It will involve speaking up, as Mother would say. And it will involve technology.

***

Back home, one spring Saturday, my weekend attendant, Richard, is pushing me through Central Park when a chance encounter changes everything. We run into two girls I know from school. They're seniors while I'm a junior, but they seem genuinely fond of me and smile pleasantly at the serendipitous meeting.

"We were just talking about you," giggles Jane.

She's in jeans and a maroon T-shirt, looking . . . comfortable. Andrea, beside her, in slightly more threadbare-and-baggy jeans and Oxford cloth, appears a shade more preppy. Both girls are tall and slender, soft-spoken and smart. I can't decide which I have a crush on. Both, probably. I have many crushes.

Distant tom-toms reverberate through the trees, giving the scene a vaguely tropical beat. I reply something stupid. Jane comes back with, "We've decided you're going to Harvard and will write for the *New Yorker*!"

A humid moment passes while I digest this. "That'll be the day," I say, echoing a popular Linda Ronstadt song of the time, and smiling involuntarily.

Afterward, something within me shifts. Ivy League nerdiness suddenly doesn't sound so bad. Yet later still, as I struggle that evening to have Richard get me comfortable in my pajamas in my wheelchair, the enormous compliment goes sour. Jane and Andrea were clearly forgetting something. They were forgetting how beset I am with the basic trivia of coping.

Or does that make any difference?

***

Around this time—1978 and '79—Mother and her friends are abuzz about two hit movies: *Coming Home* and *An Unmarried Woman*. To hear Mother talk about them, these are the most important entertainments since Erica Jong's *Fear of Flying* five years earlier!

Of course, I haven't read or seen any of them, and I won't (at least not for several more years). Not my style. I'm mystified by the smattering of sanctimoniousness I overhear about female independence and Vietnam vets and Jane Fonda. Yet what *An Unmarried Woman* means to feminism ("women's lib," in those days), *Coming Home* will come to represent for people like me.

It's not just about vets and the ravages of war. In *Coming Home*, a paralyzed vet played by a buff Jon Voight seduces the unhappy wife played by Jane Fonda—fucks her like she's never been fucked. From his wheelchair. (Okay, he transfers himself into bed, but there's a lot of lovemaking on wheels, too.)

If the Jill Clayburgh classic says *You Don't Need A Man*, the Voight-Fonda hookup shows *People In Wheelchairs Can Be Sexy*. More than that, it's the way Voight tells Fonda how to deal with him. What he needs. Instead of the usual portrayal of the self-hating cripple who can only be saved by the love of a good woman. So it's not just that those with disabilities should be welcomed and respected and loved in *all* the same ways as everybody else; it's a seismic shift in the balance of power. Because ultimately Fonda doesn't rescue him. If anything, it is *he* who rescues *her* from her miserable life with an abusive, emotionally scarred husband. Fonda is neither Voight's nurse nor his caretaker. And she is definitely not a saint for befriending him.

***

When the time comes, I do my best to type my college applications myself. I have an electric typewriter I was given for my bar mitzvah, ostensibly to exercise my fingers. Gingerly walking said fingers over the keyboard, I type slowly, carefully. Which means I'm economical in my choice of words. Mother says she'll help if needed. But I have to try to do it myself first. She's good about setting limits like that.

She's been working at Western Publishing Company, editing cook books in the Women's Division or something. She is actually a good editor with a sharp eye. She knows, for instance, that the degree my father earned at Harvard (it's on the applications, under family history) was an AB, not a BA.

The personal essay is where I think I will shine. My SAT scores are so-so, my grades are all right, but Steiner doesn't offer AP classes and I haven't achieved anything extraordinary (though I do co-edit Steiner's literary anthology and newspaper). I am, however, confident in my writing skills. My plan is to tailor one basic essay—a mixture of mild self-reflection and dollops of charm and wit—to fit each application's precise requirements. When the topic begins to take shape, it seems an obvious choice. *My Life in a Wheelchair—A unique perspective on developing character and coping skills.*

Sure. The usual bullshit. It's what people want to hear about anyway—*how do you do it? How do you manage? What's it like to be you?*

Best of all: No research necessary. No fact-checking to gum up my narrative. No one can question my authority.

A first draft flows easily. I focus on how TV- and comic-book-fueled fantasies "suffused my relationships with the physical world." From the Mighty Thor to Captain Kirk and, perhaps especially, Chief Ironside, I've spent much of my life "identifying with embattled overachievers. Is it escapism because I can't face my own reality? Perhaps. But there is more to it," I propose.

My larger-than-life heroes, trapped in alien and sometimes hostile worlds "as our barrier-laden society often seems to me," I write, "invariably prove themselves to be smarter, braver, and stronger than people expect. They give me hope and a model for patience and self-determination that I strive to emulate."

Lots of SAT words in there. But I'm particularly proud of the line: "Then adolescence struck, and I'll never forgive it!"

It's the same sort of blend of fearless honesty and beguiling nonchalance I wielded in my open letter to school from the hospital. It worked before, so why not again?

But face-to-face contact—when the admissions gatekeepers actually see me, wheels and all—may undermine the whole charade.

***

I first talk to the woman from Harvard on the phone. Kenny holds the kitchen receiver to my ear. She is a local alumna. We try to figure out how I'll get into her Brooklyn brownstone. She decides she'll come to me.

This is great! I'm thinking. Who else has the advantage of being interviewed in the comfort of home? Another benefit of being handicapped. Plus it would be foolish to dress up in one's home, right? So I don't have to go through the wardrobe agonies!

On the evening in question, Richard—my weekend attendant, who sometimes moonlights on weeknights—opens the door when she rings. A broad-shouldered, somber woman in a severe dark blue dress and pearls, she has just come from work, she says.

I offer her a drink, as I've been trained a host should do. She has no coat to hang up, or I'd have offered that first. Would've asked Richard to take it, to be precise, since I couldn't actually take it myself. I prefer thinking of my attendants as butlers or valets. They work for me, I'll say, rather than take care of me. And they are never, never nurses.

"Awfully muggy out there," says the alumna pleasantly. "Just some water, please."

"You mean we can't wine and dine you?" says Richard, suddenly chortling.

My eyes dart to my soon-to-be interlocutor. (Sorry—SAT word.) She smiles at Richard's jest, thankfully, and shakes her head. I relax into an easy camaraderie.

And this time I remember my fourth killer question:

"What sort of candidate do you think makes the ideal Harvard student? Or, to put it another way, for what sort of kids is Harvard looking?"

***

Richard is often jokey, except when he's in a mood. The first time he dressed me, I remember his quip as he closed my jeans—"So . . . should I zip up your personality?"

It seemed hilariously funny and offbeat. "Never heard it called *that* before," I said after recovering my breath.

"The older I get," he said, "the more it rings true. Your personality hangs between your legs."

I'd rather have the jokiness than the mood. The pissed-off mood. Over the years, attendants' moods will weigh heavily on me.

There's an edginess to this particular bit of humor. Mother says Richard is probably homosexual, but maybe it's just that he's from St. Louis. Being gay is a big deal in those days—considered menacing, even pre-AIDS. Mother isn't worried, though, she says, because she doesn't think I'll be easily "turned" at this point. Apparently she's worried about that before. I've never worried about *that*, but years later I'll have similar concerns, particularly in the first days of a new attendant, when I'm essentially presenting myself naked in bed to a stranger. Later still, I'll think of the gay/LGBT/queer rights movement as roughly akin to disability rights—a newly defined minority group made up largely of people intrinsically different from their own parents, who struggle in similar ways to "come out" and gain respect for just being who and what they are.

It is with Richard that I will get drunk for the first time. The attendant is not, after all, my parent or guardian (though some will think of themselves this way). It is possible for a disabled boy to be as naughty as any other boy, to keep secrets from parents, provided there's assistance from a willing helper.

Afterward, dizzy from having gulped a Black Russian like it was a milkshake, I meet Dad and Barbara at a midtown restaurant. They don't seem to notice how woozy and out of control I feel. I know I'm good at pretending but begin to wonder if they're just not that observant.

***

The anxious months of waiting for college decisions pass in a kind of preternatural calm. I become socially fearless. On weekends, with Richard's aid, I join groups of guys for smokes and sometimes beer (the weekends I'm not at Dad and Barbara's, that is). Either the guys come by my place and then wheel me across the street to the steps of the Natural History Museum—where, obviously, they park me at the bottom and perch themselves on low steps—or Richard finagles my chair into a Checker cab and deposits me at someone else's place for a few hours. My cutoff is eleven-thirty, when Richard has to bring me home and get me ready for bed, before he can go home himself. Or if I'm out with the gang, I must make sure they bring me home by then.

All of which is by way of impressing the point that, contrary to common lore, a kid in a wheelchair integrated in a regular high school class *can* fit in, *will* have friends, and is rarely subject to undue teasing. I'm sure bad things happen in some places, but by and large that's not been my experience.

Once a pal named Billy, whom I don't know that well (he's a grade or two below me), wants me to buy the beer. "I can pay for it and push you in," he explains, "but you won't get carded, man."

"I'm not eighteen."

"Does that matter?"

He's right. I've never been carded. Another benefit of being handicapped. Instant college admission, automatic permission to drink, presumed innocence even if you're guilty.

Unfortunately, these privileges don't apply to sex.

I ask girls out every now and then. We'll meet at a restaurant on Columbus Avenue or a movie—I figure they can push my chair a little ways if necessary. Somehow, though, I steer clear of actually having a girlfriend. I tell myself it's because I'm not trying hard enough, or not settling for less than perfection. I never once think no girl will have me because of my disability.

At a friend's party one night, I begin kissing a girl who was always just a good friend before. Or maybe she starts kissing me. It goes on a long, luscious time, but only so far. I don't notice or understand when something changes. Maybe a neighbor complains about the noise. Whatever the cause, the party is abruptly over. I ask someone to call Richard, tell him to pick me up. The interlude is never mentioned again.

But over spring break, another female school friend visits. We're supposed to rehearse lines for the class play. Unbelievably, there's a button missing from her blouse. Soon all her buttons are open and she has no bra. I haven't liked her in that way before, but hey—tits! I'm in my motorized wheelchair, and drive myself close to where she's sitting. From that vantage point, I'm able to reach a hand over and feel her breasts. But I don't really know what to do with my fingers. We kiss with tongues, which feels nicer than I would have thought, but then she winces. "Your fingers are cold," she says. The phone rings, and Richard—oblivious at the other end of the apartment—says it's Dad. After the phone call, the lusty mood is broken. Though she is willing to continue, I say no. It just doesn't feel right.

Soon she's on her way home, both of us confused. I can't help noticing that my social life wouldn't be possible if Dad hadn't moved out and Mother weren't engaged in an active social life herself.

That is, when she's not sick in bed all weekend from radiation and chemo.

***

I get in every college I applied to, with one exception: Yale, my favorite, where I'm wait-listed.

An agony of indecision ensues—until it dawns on me. Like it or not, for better or worse, to have Harvard on my résumé will serve me well. Especially since I'm not naturally gifted with scholarly talents. Or perhaps because a guy in a wheelchair needs all the credibility, the merit badges, he can muster. Not that the same couldn't be said of any of the other fine schools. But Harvard seems the prototype. The original. Plus I can picture a sort of punk rock cool to being an iconoclast among the ancient bricks and ivy.

Those are the only terms under which I will go. I will not choose Harvard to uphold a family tradition. I'll go in my own way. If I think about it at all, I suppose it doesn't hurt that Alec is there in case I ever need help.

So that summer, Dad starts talking to Harvard about my specific access requirements. At fifty-three, Dad still likes solving problems—or rather, he doesn't accept a degree of blind faith, of unresolved mystery, which is all I've got to rely on when it comes to gauging how I'm going to cope at Harvard.

"No idea," I say, when Dad looks at me for reassurance about how I'll manage. "But I've always coped before somehow, and somehow I'll do it again."

Per my parents' divorce agreement, I spend about half the summer at Dad and Barbara's. The house they moved to in Stamford to raise Jeff is a big two-story with four bedrooms. Three stories, if you count the finished basement. They installed a small elevator for me.

Also per the divorce agreement, Dad takes over primary custody of me after high school. Which shouldn't mean anything to me—mostly has to do with financial arrangements between my estranged parents—but it does. It sits heavy in my gut. I'm Dad's now.

What's worse, I'm spending extra weekends here while Mother undergoes more radiation treatments. For some time now she's been wearing weird wigs. She hopes no one notices, and I hope so too, though for different reasons. It seems almost weirder to have a mother who wears a wig than to have one who has cancer!

***

One weekend Dad and I visit Cambridge. We meet Thomas Crooks, the Dean of Harvard College—a tall man with a warm, syrupy voice who looks precisely as you'd expect. Pipe-smoking, dressed all in tweed with elbow patches, even on a warm summer afternoon. He'll become my main contact point at Harvard for issues involving accessibility, though he's not actually a user—that is, not disabled—himself.

Crooks introduces us to Will, a graduate student he's appointed to oversee handicapped undergrads, a new position born of recent federal regulations. He's not handicapped either.

Still, Will is likable—a blond, curly-haired, energetic camp-counselor-type. As he demonstrates the college's new lift-equipped van and a modern freshman dorm called Canaday—which has two ground-floor, wheelchair-accessible suites, each with a big living room and either two or three adjacent bedrooms (one of which could be filled by a live-in attendant)—I remain guarded. I've always preferred taking my disability in stride, getting by by winging it, not by taking a cold hard look at my limitations or needs. Certainly never explaining them to others. How the hell should I know how many inches wide my big motorized wheelchair is?

Throughout the trip Dad is jovial and proud. Lots of handshaking, pats on the back, and Harvardian camaraderie. Not sure I want to be a member of the order, but my sense is they are damn proud of it and absolutely confident that Harvard will do the right thing. Later, I will write about these first encounters in the student weekly newsmagazine, the *Harvard Independent*:

> People seemed interested and enthusiastic about having a student like me. The place was willing, but the works remained practically untried.

. . . I am not afraid of a school designed for the ambulatory. But I was planning to live on campus; frankly, I was anxious about how a college, especially a Harvard, could effectively accommodate me. Let's face it: this place is old. It's full of cracks and bumps and stairs . . .

[I soon learned] the University was busy planning for my arrival. I was phoned by the Freshman Dean Office [*sic.*] for the dimensions of my widest and heaviest wheelchair. As the summer progressed, I found myself engaged more than once in conversations with the FDO, particularly with Will . . ., a senior adviser. We discussed every aspect of my life (and I mean *every*).

I was forced to consider questions I couldn't begin to answer. Daily activities I had never thought twice about before were suddenly objects of scrutiny. How big should a bathroom be? Did I really need a tub or would the shower do? Could I open the front door to my suite by myself? The future was nebulous; all I could do was guess at the answers.

When we circle back to Crooks' office, two disappointments undermine the conviviality. First, we're told that the extra bedroom in the accessible suite, for my live-in attendant, won't come free; Dad will have to pay for it, too. Second, I can't have a roommate, just the attendant.

"I'm confused," I stammer.

"We don't want to put any undue burden on other students, whether explicitly or implicitly," explains Henry Moses, another dean. "Perhaps when you're a sophomore . . . "

Never mind any undue burden on *me*. The burden of isolation.

***

Before Labor Day, Dad puts an ad in the *Boston Globe* for attendants. We figure one live-in during the week and another on weekends. I've never had a live-in attendant before. I wish Kenny could move with me but his wife's just had a baby.

Again, my mantra: Somehow I'll manage. I've always coped before against unlikely odds.

The first candidate we interview on a subsequent visit to Cambridge is a man in his thirties, an aspiring cellist. Dad likes him and doesn't understand when I say, afterward, "Yes, but he'd be working for *me*, not you."

My favorite candidate shows up later—a Harvard junior planning to take the next year off. His name is Michael. Tall, dark-haired, personable, he smiles a lot and seems to get my jokes. I think we could be buddies. That's good enough for me. I don't consider why he's taking the next year off.

In the final days of summer I get my first new motorized wheelchair in more than seven years. It's supposed to be tough enough for cobblestones and snow, and I intend to use it all the time, not just indoors. Which is something I think I've been wanting a long time but wasn't technologically practical before. The obvious negatives are, it doesn't fold up into a car trunk and is too heavy to lift up steps without a team of strong men. There are, I will discover, less obvious negatives, too.

When the big day comes, Dad arrives at the Beresford with a U-Haul attached to the lumbering Checker. He loads it while Mother fusses about what not to forget. It's hot and humid and Dad's sweating profusely. Mother's bugging him about carefully stowing my precious possessions, and I can see Dad's going to lose his temper. What I can't determine is whose side to take.

Finally Dad gets me and the new electric wheelchair. Mom waves from the corner and I stare out the window. It will be the last time I see her standing.

CHAPTER SIX

MAMAN EST MORTE

1980-1981

"What makes you a writer? You develop an extra sense that partly excludes you from experience."
—Martin Amis, in *The Paris Review*, Spring 1998

Before Columbus Day weekend, when freshman parents visit, Alec calls to pass on a message from Bob. Mother isn't well and might not be able to visit Harvard after all.

"I'm sorry, Ben. But *I* could visit you."

I'm listening to him through my new speakerphone. The phone company has supplied me with one just like the one I saw in Berkeley. I have to dial out to make calls, using a regular touch-tone phone, and then transfer the call to speaker, but I can easily tap the remote button to answer when the phone rings. I keep a list of important numbers next to the phone and speaker setup. The list includes several home-health-care agencies with winning names like "Quality Care" that make me never want to call them, ever.

Though he's only a few streets away, in Lowell House, Alec and I have scarcely seen each other since I've been here. And then it was accidental. He's never had a sense of responsibility for me, and I've never wanted to have that kind of relationship with him. Decades later I'll realize that he's never helped feed me or taken me to the bathroom.

In the vastness of Harvard, I figure he's giving me my space as much as he may be preserving his own.

"'S'okay," I say. "Just wonder why Bob called *you*, not me."

"Bob's a boob."

"Yes. Bob's a boob." Then something occurs to me and I add, "Should we do something? For Mother, I mean."

Long pause. In my mind I'm going through the possibilities . . . send a get-well card? Call on the phone? Surely not send flowers!

"How the fuck should I know? Boob didn't say anything like that. He just wanted you to know about Freshman Parents' Weekend."

"Why didn't he just call me, then?"

"Why do you ask stupid questions? I guess he called me because I'm the Big Buzzy!"

That's our old childhood slang for him. Short for "big brother." And I was Little Benjie.

Privately, I take it back. He *has* felt responsible for me. But in a patronizing way, nothing practical or helpful. So I tease, to bring him down a peg. I tease and he curses. Then we both curse and tease. This is the pattern with us. Even now, neither of us talks about Mother's health. We both know what's going on, so why talk about it?

The next day Bob calls me. Maybe Alec told him to, or maybe Bob decided he doesn't like using Alec as messenger. They've never gotten along very well. "Your mother wants to visit you," he says. "She probably shouldn't, but anyway, I'm going with her, to help out. All right?"

Yes. Of course. But it's a rhetorical question, right? What's he really asking me?

"Ben, your mother is having a lot of difficulties. I don't want you to worry—*she* doesn't want you to worry—but you understand? This is from the cancer."

"Mm-hmm."

"Just thought you should understand. Before you see her. "

After we hang up I call Alec, but no one answers. I should let him know what Bob said—that Mom is coming up after all but isn't well. I wonder if I'll remember to call Alec again later. I wonder why Bob is so worried. Mom has had cancer for three years now. She's had bad spells before. She always bounces back. We're pretty used to it.

Nothing to worry about.

***

When they arrive, Mom can scarcely walk by herself and leans on Bob for every step. She smiles wanly when we make eye contact, struggles to bend down to kiss my cheek, and then has to sit down. We go inside my dorm suite.

I don't think we've ever sat across a table from each other like this just to talk. We've always been an integral part of each other's daily lives, ever in the background or foreground, never so separate as to need to catch up. She's moving like an old lady yet somehow I am unable to see her that way. She still looks well put together, just tired or weak or clumsy. Have days like that myself.

Too long a quiet moment passes. What on earth should we talk about?

Another, more chilling question courses through me: Should I ask about her health? Wouldn't that be the mature, polite thing to do? Yet that would mean that I noticed. I think she's trying to pretend things are fine. There's a line I feel forbidden to cross. Like a big pimple on someone's face or a piece of spinach stuck between a companion's teeth—glaringly obvious, rude to call attention to. I let her lead, and it becomes clear that her health is the last thing she wants to talk about. With me anyway.

"Aren't you cold?" she says.

"No, Mom. A little, but I'm fine. Autumn in Massachusetts."

I called her "Mom" instead of "Mother."

She wants to hear about what I'm doing. I talk randomly about my classes. I do not complain. The classes are large and difficult and I feel lost in the crowd. It's not easy getting around such a large campus in a wheelchair. I have to preregister for classes, to make sure the ones I want are held in or moved to accessible locations. One Shakespeare class can't be moved, so I'm taking it at night, through the extension school but for regular credit. In addition, the ubiquitous bricks and cobblestones of Cambridge are bumpy. I'm using my motorized wheelchair full time now, yet still usually have my new, live-in attendant Michael or a volunteer from the fledgling Disabled Students Office follow along just in case. I miss WNEW-FM, my New York indie rock station. And my old, trusted attendants Kenny and Richard. And the thrum of life in New York, the center of the world. But if any such remark accidentally slips I reflexively follow it with "but I'm coping" or "but it's getting better" or "but I've been through worse." I'm used to reassuring others about my well being. I'm usually more honest with Mom but here, now, she's just another person.

After a short time she has to lie down.

***

The first time she mentioned her cancer to us was just before my first hospitalization. When I was in ninth grade, Alec in eleventh. I remember how she tried to sound very serious. Alec and I must have looked like we didn't care, like we had better things to do. Mother often had serious talks with us about things that were on her mind—drugs, birth control—that never actually cropped up as true problems for us. So why take her seriously now? Such was my adolescent logic.

What happened in the three years since then was largely kept in the background. Here's what we did know: Her hair fell out and she wore wigs. We were not to talk about her "illness" with others, especially not her colleagues at Western Publishing Company. "Why is it a secret?" I wanted to know.

"People might have funny reactions," she said. "I'll let them know when I'm ready."

She did her research, trying to pick the best oncologist in New York. She kept a diary of the ordeal, was going to turn it into a book, she said. I still have the hundred or so pages of manuscript she did manage to complete—along with notes scribbled on scraps of paper and cocktail napkins, and memos from her agent urging her to get the damn thing done. Mother was a procrastinator, but then, how would *you* spend your final months on earth? At the typewriter or out in the world?

There were weekends after her treatments that she spent entirely locked in her bedroom. That's partly why she hired Richard more. She hired Richard to stay overnight to take care of me. She was not to be disturbed. Once, though, when her door was open a crack, I saw her rushing, stooped over, from her bed for the toilet to throw up.

And another time we invaded her sanctum because it had the only cable TV in the house. She seemed fine about it—it was Sunday evening, and the nausea had mostly passed. Then I heard her on the phone with Bob. "Can't you do something to help me? Something useful and constructive? Why? You ask me why? Because it hurts. I'm hurting. Do you understand?"

I pretended not to hear.

***

A few nights after Mother's visit I wake up and call out to Michael. I need to change my position in bed. My legs are stiff and my left knee hurts from pressing on the mattress too long in one position. It's routine, happens two or three times most nights. We've strung an intercom between our two bedrooms, a sort of baby monitor, just in case. But this night I call and holler and shout and he doesn't respond. I listen to see if I can hear him snoring or anything else that might clue me in. My left knee especially is hurting.

Using my stomach muscles, such as they are, I'm able to shake myself on the bed just enough to alleviate the painful pressure temporarily. But the relief is so short-lived, so ineffectual, I become even more frustrated. The pain grows unbearable—made worse by the knowledge that it could be eliminated so easily. WHERE IS HE? I shout out again and again until I don't know what else to do. Eventually, begrudgingly, I must fall back to sleep because the next thing I know it's morning and he's there.

I wait until he's gotten me safely dressed and in my chair before broaching the subject. "You certainly slept soundly last night, yeah?" I half-ask, half-accuse.

"Not really." He chuckles in an aw-shucks manner. "I can't stop yawning this morning—"

"Because you didn't hear me last night when I called you."

He acts completely surprised. "What? No. I—you—when?"

"I couldn't see the clock but it was my usual leg-turning—I called and called!"

"I'm sorry," he says, grinning nervously. "Um, I did go out briefly. Had to run to the library for a book. It was only a moment."

I'm stunned, filled with fear-squelching hostility. He went out? He actually left me alone in the middle of the night? And surely it was longer than a *moment*. Left me in bed where I can't do anything, can't even get to the phone. I could be left alone sitting at my table, set up with a book or the electric typewriter. But not in bed. It's my most vulnerable . . . Who would do something like that? Surely I've explained this to him before. Surely it's . . . it's unthinkable! Such negligence!

"You can't disappear when I'm in bed," I come back confidently. I hope I sound confident. I emphasize how immobile I am in bed. "Can't even reach the phone," I say. "Can I rely on you from now on?"

He nods, mumbles an apology. "I didn't know—"

"This must never happen again."

I'm tough. But I know there's nothing I can do to stop him if he does disappear again. And I realize my life is now in the hands of someone I don't trust.

***

To get to the basement office of the *Harvard Independent*, the student newsweekly, I have to get into my old manual wheelchair and be carried down a steep flight of steps. It's easy enough to recruit muscular young guys eager to show off, but I'm not exactly comfortable being jostled by a wolf pack of strangers. I only visit the office once—on Comp Night, when the rules of the competition to be accepted on staff are explained. This is the way extracurricular activities work at Harvard. Everything is a competition.

There are snacks on a side table—well, bags of Doritos. I love Doritos but I've come without my attendant and there's no table to pull into, no place high enough to put Doritos within my reach. So when offered I say no thanks. I say I had a big lunch. There are limits to how much help I'm willing to ask of strangers.

Actually, I can't even decide if the problem is in me—my shyness, my physical disability itself—or something external . . . something to do with inadequate access. So I relegate Unscheduled Snacking to the category of Spontaneous Activities From Which I Must Abstain, and soldier on.

My first submission is a long feature about Harvard's efforts to comply with new accessibility regulations. It's accepted, published in a big two-page spread. It begins:

> In the midst of the academic year and the deadlines that go with it, Harvard students—especially freshmen, who are faced with some new Core regulations—may feel frustrated, picked on, or even downright small. But the University has some new requirements to meet, too. As of September 1980, all school programs must have been made accessible to handicapped persons. With a campus as old as Harvard's, this is certainly a challenging task, if not an outright impossibility. But a wheel-chair bound student can negotiate Harvard more easily than you might imagine. I know—I'm one, and I've been getting along fine.

Typically upbeat and breezy. Call it a puff piece, but I know how to please my audience.

This becomes my first experience as a sort of freelancer—writing stories in my dorm room and having someone else deliver them. My only interaction being by telephone. Not bad but I know I'll never be a fully integrated member of the staff, never enjoy the heady camaraderie of teamwork, simply because the office is out of bounds for the "wheelchair-bound." It occurs to me now that this is the kind of frustration I'd never admit in those days, even in an article about campus accessibility.

Still, I like writing—proud to be published on my first try, proud to have strangers stop me in the Yard to say, "Are you the guy who wrote that great article?"—and publish a few more pieces, even one cartoon. Quickly, though, the sense of being unwelcome, of being an outsider, grows burdensome. I tell my editor I've simply become too busy to keep up a regular flow of articles. Besides, I discover I'm not cut out to be a roving reporter. The Harvard campus is too big and inaccessible for that. So I quit the paper.

***

Three weeks before my eighteenth birthday, Ronald Reagan is elected president (for the first time). I can't vote, but if I could I probably would've voted for him. I say probably because everyone I know seems to think that's a bad idea. But I like Ronnie. I like the Republican ideal of self-determination. I certainly haven't survived by whining and feeling sorry for myself, and the last thing I need is government pity. I also kind of relate to Reagan's movie-soaked vision of the world, his devotion to fantasy to determine the best course of action. It's always worked for *me*.

Soon, however, the Reagan Administration will seek to revoke equal-access regulations as acts of Big Government that fetter economic expansion by unfairly burdening the private sector and taxpayers. I would feel betrayed if I were paying any attention to politics.

One evening I'm heading to dinner in the Freshman Union, with Michael following behind—to be precise, we're going through the separate wheelchair-accessible entrance. A passing fellow Canaday resident sees us and blurts, "I'll see you later. Nine o'clock, right?"

Puzzled, I notice Michael is waving his arms frantically. The other guy suddenly glows red. I roll onto the wheelchair lift, wait for Michael to push the button. I wonder what he's up to. What's at nine o'clock?

I no longer trust Michael. But I can't confront him now. I want my dinner.

Yet as we enter the dining hall, I can no longer control myself. In the safety of the crowd, I ask him about that strange little conversation outside.

"Don't make me tell you," he says.

I get angrier and angrier—borderline accusatory—until he finally caves. The truth: He's throwing me a surprise birthday party. He has conspired with Alec, who doesn't know about the other night, to host it tonight in Canaday's Common Room.

I know I should be relieved. Flattered, even. But my attitude toward Michael has soured, so nothing feels right.

"I've got work to do," I say, unconsciously channeling Chief Ironside grumpiness again, like in fifth grade. "And I don't like surprises!"

He begs me to go along, for the sake of everybody involved. So I do. I do not believe this is why he disappeared the other night—and he doesn't pretend it is. I'm still angry and scared. And suspicious. Is he trying to appease me, to distract me from his shortcomings?

Still, the party *is* a blast. The entire section of our dorm is there, along with a few other friends I've made plus Alec and his new girlfriend. I'm given an old Who album, the new John Lennon record *Double Fantasy*, and a Harvard piggy bank that still sits on my shelf today.

Alec and I haven't spent any time together since Freshman Parents' Weekend more than a month ago. I'm glad to see him though I haven't missed him. He's got his own, established cadre of brainy Lowell House friends while I'm trying to develop a hipper niche. Hipper in theory, anyway.

It's not entirely true that our paths haven't crossed, however. A couple of times we've spotted each other across the Yard or tooling down Mount Auburn Street. But we've exchanged few words. It usually goes something like this:

"Hey, Asshole!" he bellows at me with a big smile and wave.

"It's the faggot!" I reply.

Laugh. Smile.

"How's your ass?"

"Smaller than yours, freak!"

"Suck my dick!"

"Fuck you!"

I can't yell as loudly as he does. Nevertheless, Alec guffaws at the top of his robust voice, so everyone in a hundred-mile radius can hear.

"Who is that, cursing you out?" asks a concerned passing stranger.

"My brother," I answer.

The stranger looks confused. And I realize I am, too. Why is this what my relationship with Alec has become?

***

Thanksgiving weekend, Michael comes home to New York with me. His family is in Colorado, too far to visit. Mother insists on hosting Turkey Day at our place just like she's always done, only this time Bob has hired a couple of caterers to cook and serve and clean up. Mother is trying to pretend everything is normal.

In December Michael has more absences. Things start disappearing from my room. One evening I accuse him. I'm unrelenting, and he starts to cry. He swears he has not stolen from me, but confesses he has disappeared at night many times when I'm asleep. He goes out to drink, do drug deals, or meet the blonde girl from upstairs to share a few joints and screw on the Canaday Common Room sofa.

"I'm no good," he says in tearful gasps. "All right? I admit it! I'm a liar and an alcoholic and I like drugs! I probably should be thrown out of Harvard . . . and would have been if I didn't take this year off. But I don't steal. I didn't take your stuff!"

I tell him he's betrayed my trust and he has to make it up to me. I give him another chance. After all, what are my alternatives? I have the phone numbers of a half-dozen home-care agencies but they're expensive and it's impossible to find a good male attendant. I don't have a better backup plan. God, I wish Kenny could've come up here with me!

A few nights later John Lennon is gunned down. The Dakota is just blocks from the Beresford, my childhood home. I have a fantasy that I should have been there. This will be my generation's Kennedy Moment, an instant frozen in memory forever.

At lunch the next day (I never go for breakfast), the Freshman Union is eerily quiet. The student body is in mourning. The radio stations play nothing but John and Beatles music all day, even bootlegs. That night there is a TV special about his life. I want to watch it. Michael has something else scheduled but promises to be back in time to turn on the TV for me. He is not.

***

Fred, one of my weekend attendants, comes with me to New York over Christmas break. He stays in Mother's bedroom because she's not there. She's at Bob's apartment on Fifth Avenue. Fred walks with me through Central Park to visit her. It's freezing outside, and Bob's place feels warm and bright.

In the month since Thanksgiving, Mother has been living in a rented hospital bed in his dining room. Bob has hired a full-time nurse—an efficient older woman with an adorable Irish accent. I'm sorry to have forgotten her name now.

Fred and I settle in Bob's living room. There's a breathtaking view of Central Park, the trees bald and stark in the winter light. Mother is escorted in, shaky in a pink and blue nightgown. The nurse leads her to a high-backed soft chair near where I've parked. Mother can reach my knee and pats it. A ghostly smile brightens her drawn face. She is at once wan and—to me, at least—luminous. She holds my hand and asks to hear about how I'm doing. I look at her hard, then look down. She's thin and gray, her skin transparent.

As at her Cambridge visit, I prattle on about all the good things. I talk with intensity, with a sense of wonder at what's different in my new life. Not the bad stuff, of course—all the while aware that my life is expanding while hers closes in.

I go on too long, though my exact words are meaningless and quickly forgotten. Mother never interrupts or contributes except to nod occasionally or blink her full-moon eyes. After forty-five minutes the nurse reappears.

"Mrs. Mattlin—uh, your mom—needs to rest now."

I smile. She helps Mother stand. Mother touches me on the head as she shambles past. Fred, who has been quiet throughout, rises like a Marine at attention and abruptly is at my side. He is short, and I can feel his breath on my hair.

At the elevator Fred asks, "What's wrong? What's she got?"

"Cancer." My one-word answer. I don't want to talk about it.

People have asked versions of the same question about *me* so many times I find that I have no patience for it. Does the precise diagnosis really matter? Besides, doesn't Fred already know my mother has cancer? It seems like everybody must know by now! In my world it's a big event.

***

By the end of 1980, the United Nations has designated the following year to be the first International Year of Disabled Persons. Already grassroots advocacy campaigns are springing up in far-flung places, such as Singapore's Disabled Peoples' International. And in Louisville, Kentucky, a young activist-journalist named Mary Johnson launches a newsletter about the budding disability-rights movement called the *Disability Rag*, which will become an unofficial lodestar. Within a few years the *Rag* will be written up in the *Wall Street Journal* in an article Dad will send me—an article that will open me to a new consciousness about "disability culture."

The press also alerts the world to atrocious abuse that's going on in the nation's nursing homes. In 1980, Congress passes the Civil Rights of Institutionalized Persons Act authorizing the Justice Department to file civil suits on behalf of residents whose rights are being violated. The campaign continues even today.

Make no mistake: The world's consciousness of the rights of and injustices toward disabled people is being raised in many ways. Yet I stay out of that orbit. I'm too busy coping with my own crises.

***

After New Year's comes finals. Back in Cambridge, I fire Michael and hire a new weekday attendant on my own, having watched Dad do the interviewing before. (Fred still comes on weekends but can only stay during the week for a short time.) You sort of prompt each applicant to fill in the blanks of their lives, like helping them put together a résumé, in a way, which none of them actually has. You always get two or three references and, as a last step, interview the references over the phone.

The new attendant, Tom, is blond, blue-eyed, and in his early thirties. Recently returned to Boston after a stint in the Army, Tom is a bit of a rough-

and-tumble guy who smokes cigarettes, and I like the smell. I'm in a hurry to find someone, and he seems the best candidate because he's quiet, orderly, responsible. He arrives at his interview on time and has decent references. Admittedly not much to go on.

There's another school break after finals. Tom comes with me on the train to New York. One evening I go out with old high school friends and when they bring me home I have to wake Tom up. It's only nine-thirty and he's fallen asleep in what used to be Mother's bed. I ask him for a glass of orange juice. He says okay and I wait. I sit at the dinner table and wait and wait and call him again. Alec is there but he doesn't do anything. Tom finally comes stumbling into the room and says, "What?"

"Orange juice, please."

"All right! All right! I'm not your fuckin' nigger, you know!"

I say, "Just wake up, man."

(Tom is White.)

He gets the orange juice and then stumbles to the bathroom. Alec comes in, looks at me with his mouth open. He's heard the whole thing.

The next day Bob takes the three of us to lunch at his favorite restaurant, *Les Pleiades*, on Seventy-fifth near Madison. When Tom gets up to use the men's room, Alec tells Bob what happened last night. "Does he look hung-over to you?" Alec asks.

"No. It's not something you can tell by looking," says Bob.

"He says he was just sleeping," I offer optimistically.

Tom returns. After lunch we go back to Bob's, which is just around the corner, and spend a few minutes with Mother. This time she doesn't even get out of the hospital bed. She tries to reach me through the side rail but mostly can only touch me with her eyes.

A few weeks later I have to tell Tom to leave. He's had other drunk episodes. I make sure Fred is with me when I lower the ax, for my own protection.

Tom doesn't protest much or make excuses. He packs a bag and evaporates.

Desperate, I call a home-health-care agency. It's really a nurses' registry but I explain that I'm not sick, I'm not a patient, I don't need a nurse. The woman on the phone still doesn't understand or can't believe I'm calling for myself. "And who are *you*?" she asks me twice, as if I must be the parent or spouse of the person I'm calling about. Of the "patient," as she says.

She uses words like *CNA* and *LVN* and *aid*. These refer to levels of training, I quickly discern. I explain the tasks and let her determine the appropriate level for me.

Fred is able to stay overnight. In the morning a large cheerful man from the agency appears. His name is Bill, and he's a bit of a matronly aunt—in manner and speech, I mean . . . perhaps I should say a *"bearded* aunt," since his face is dominated by a full red beard and glasses. He is in surgical scrubs, but I like him. He's not cool like Kenny but he's alert and bright and responsible and understands the job at hand.

In the spare bedroom in my Canaday suite, Bill finds Tom's leftover chicken bones hiding in the desk drawers, empty beer bottles and cans under the bed, and cigarette butts everywhere. "Oh my, oh my! I *must* give this room a thorough cleaning ova!" he declares in his Bostonian brogue.

After a few days Bill suggests a deal. He'll stay on as my live-in attendant during the week but not tell the agency. "You'll save money—or should I say your dad will save money—and I'll make more," he explains. "You see? Simple."

***

The summer after my freshman year at Harvard, Bill agrees to stay in New York with me. One day in early June we walk across Central Park to Bob's place to see Mother. The nurse greets us at the door with a long face. "I'm so sorry," she says.

I don't get it. "'S'all right," I say casually, trying to cheer her up. People have been sorry for me too many times.

Mother turns her head in bed to smile at me but this time says nothing at all. She doesn't sit up, just keeps lying there looking at me. So I talk at her.

For some reason I tell her I'm still interested in religion and how, just last night, I was reading a passage in the Torah that felt profound. It was the psalm about what is mortal man that God should be mindful of us.

I ramble on to her warm, receptive smile.

"It struck me, that's all, how fortunate we are, all of us, and how much worse things could be and perhaps should be considering how often people aren't good to one another," I say.

I expect my Tiny Tim prattle to be challenged. She doesn't speak or even change expressions. Her eyes blink, but her lips are locked in a tight smile. That's okay with me. I believe she is listening. And I mean what I've said. For me, reading Torah is going back to my roots—or my grandfathers' roots, really—something I need to do just now. Not unlike re-reading old comic books or watching *Star Trek* reruns. Comfortingly familiar, stable, unchanging. It's been rough since September. But I've survived my first year at Harvard. I'm duly proud and thankful, and wonder what right I have to express dissatisfaction, to ask for anything more.

When Mother starts to fall asleep Bill takes me home.

Alec and I have the apartment to ourselves, though Bill is in Mother's old bedroom. Our only cable TV is in there, and Alec and I stay up late watching. We watch Ugly George and *Interludes After Midnight*—local public-access porn on Channel J. Then there's some soft-core bimbo movie on HBO. When it's over we go to the kitchen to get a snack and play Crazy Eights, a childhood favorite. It, too, is like comfort food.

The doorbell rings. It must be after one in the morning. Bill gets the door and when he sees who it is he murmurs "Oh" and retires to the bedroom.

Alec and I come toward the door. It's Dad. What's he doing here at this hour?

"I'm sorry, boys," he says quietly.

Alec and I look at each other for a moment, lost, but the moment doesn't last.

"Bob called me and I came right over."

"From Stamford?" I ask.

"Yes. Bob thought perhaps I should be the one to tell you it's over. You mother is gone."

***

Dad sits with us in the living room for a long time with only a dim light on. He helps himself to Courvoisier, which he knows where to find, and offers us some. "Ever had it?" he asks. "Fire water!"

I try a sip. He's right. Fire water. We each take a glass.

"*Aujourd'hui, maman est morte*," says Alec. "'Today my mother died,'" he translates. "It's the opening of Camus' *L'Étranger*," he explains.

I'm not sure what that contributes to the conversation but I'm impressed. He really is the smart one.

After a time Dad suggests we get some sleep. He sets his tall frame down on the trundle bed in my room. I lie there not wanting to sleep. I want this day to go on. That is, I don't want to let go of it. This day Mom *was* alive at least. Tomorrow she'll have no claim on.

***

Bob makes the funeral arrangements, per Mom's wishes. Dad decides to go with us to the service and stands behind me the whole time. Somebody says there are those present who don't approve of Dad's being there. They feel he who caused my mother so much pain and sorrow should not be among those who mourn her. Dad maybe is the one who tells me this. He's braced for it. He says he's there for *us*.

The Frank Campbell Mortuary is packed. People come up to me like they know me but I don't know them. I don't have a black suit but wear my navy blazer. Dad, usually a stickler for proper dress, says it's okay.

Afterward, he lifts me into the black limo that follows the hearse to Mom's plot in Westchester County. Bob chose the cemetery and pays for it and the funeral, too. He says he asked Mom a while ago about her burial wishes and she said she just could not deal with it. She asked him to decide. She had only one condition: It should be someplace where I can visit whenever I want to. Someplace wheelchair-accessible.

During the long limo ride I feel hyper-alert. Perhaps I don't know what sorrow feels like. I believe Mom would understand. "Right behind ya, Ma," I say inside my head, thinking Mom would appreciate the little joke though I can't exactly explain it myself. It doesn't make sense, and I decide to keep it private. It's the first time I realize I'm thinking of her as "Mom" again, not "Mother." And I never go back.

It's a nice cemetery. That's what Dad and Alec say. Alec notices that Ira Gershwin is buried in a mausoleum near the entrance. Who? I think. Alec is again making it clear that he's better educated, better read, more sophisticated than I am. But then again, who gives a fuck who else is buried here? At the graveside ceremony I see one of Mom's oldest, closest friends weeping uncontrollably.

Still I do not weep.

***

Through most of the summer Mom's friends invite Alec and me to dinner. Alec has a job in the city and I'm trying to write a short story, one that's as good as a John Updike story Mom showed me in the *New Yorker* sometime ago. Some of her friends are especially concerned about me. I'm younger and was more dependent on Mom, they explain. But I'm not upset or sad, and reassure them I'm fine. Mom and I had a good connection. That last day I spoke with her about Torah. What could have been a finer farewell?

In fact, I'm unable to let sorrow interfere in my life. Sadness is too debilitating; it has been wrung out of me. Mom taught me that self-discipline, not crying or self-pity, will get me through. And I believe it's true. (Historians in the budding disability-studies discipline might call this the FDR Model of strength not through but *from* adversity.)

Austin, my old camp counselor and first male attendant, who has moved to Israel and renamed himself Avraham, sends me a book about Jewish mourning customs. I try to observe all except for the difficult ones like sitting shivah and saying kaddish at Temple every Friday night. I have no residual issues or guilt. Not like Alec.

One of the last things Alec said to her was a lie, he tells me later. He was late with his application for a summer internship and didn't want Mom to know. So he said he'd done it when he hadn't.

Later, one sentence from her funeral sticks in my brain. "This was supposed to be a wedding," says Bob, "but God had something else in mind."

———●———

CHAPTER SEVEN

WHAT I GAINED AND LOST IN COLLEGE

1982-1983

"If you have some daily anguish from some cause that's not really your fault—a rotten family, bad health, nowhere looks, serious money problems, nobody to help you, minority background (I don't have that—a WASP—but I had other things), rejoice! These things are your fuel!"
—Helen Gurley Brown, draft of
Having It All, noted in *The Late Show*

The short story I write is called "Always Fighting." It describes four events in a young man's life that should've gone more easily. The first is a childhood sunburn, which turns a pleasant day at the beach into a trauma (true story). Then comes an irreparable fight with a close friend in college (fiction), followed by the death of the young man's mother (true). In the final scene, he's lying in bed on a hot, humid summer night, unable to sleep. The air conditioner is blowing too cold. If he gets up to adjust it, he knows he'll quickly become too hot again. Those sad memories—the shadows of betrayal—rush through his mind as he reflects that life is sometimes monumentally unfair.

It takes all summer to type and re-type the twelve pages—each word (each letter, considering the way I type) painstakingly considered. Yet I cannot explain why in heck he doesn't just get up and fetch a blanket or fiddle with the thermostat. In short, I can't explain his paralysis. I say he's too exhausted and frustrated to move. But the truth is I don't dare make him handicapped like me.

Nevertheless, the story gains me entrée to a closed creative writing seminar at Harvard—one of the few classes I take as a sophomore that I actually enjoy—though I know deep inside that I haven't found my "voice," that thing everyone says you're supposed to have. For me, every phrase is measured by the yardstick of John Updike.

Emulating Updike and his ilk is nothing more than an attempt to appease Mom's ghost and win Dad's approval. And as far as I know at that point, authors in this league don't write about disabilities—except perhaps symbolically, as precursors to death and metaphors for emotional or societal damage. Tiny Tim. The Hunchback of Notre Dame. There are victims galore—cancer sufferers, blind or limping young women ripe for abuse—and demented, deformed villains such as hunchbacked Richard III or paralyzed Mrs. Clennam from *Little Dorrit*. I don't see myself in them.

To me, the best are the inspirational heroes—plucky overachievers who overcome impossible hurdles (like FDR, Chief Ironside, or the blind superhero Daredevil, say). But is there no place in educated society for someone like me—*unless* I'm an overachiever?

Where is the disabled Richard Wright or Ralph Ellison? Where is the authentic disability experience?

***

Actually, it's cropping up everywhere in various ways I just don't know about yet. The very week I finish my story, the obituary for Christy Brown appears in newspapers, on a page I never read (now the obits are one of the first sections I look at). If I had noticed, I might've remembered Mom's description of Brown a few years ago as the Irishman who painted with one foot.

Earlier that same week—on Labor Day, 1981—the *New York Times* ran an op-ed by Evan J. Kemp Jr.—a prominent Washington, DC, attorney with spinal muscular atrophy (a version of my diagnosis). He headed an advocacy group called the Disability Rights Center and, in his op-ed, calls to task the Jerry Lewis-Muscular Dystrophy Association telethon.

> "The very human desire for cures . . . can never justify a television show that reinforces a stigma against disabled people. These prejudices create stereotypes that offend our

self-respect, harm our efforts to live independent lives, and segregate us from the mainstream of society."

Kemp's words are a battle cry! A call to arms! If only I'd been paying attention.

I'll read about the no-more-pity campaign later, in the *Disability Rag.* I'll even go on to publish a related essay in the *Los Angeles Times* a decade later. And toward the end of his too-short life, Kemp will launch a publishing enterprise that will become my first regular (part-time) employer.

In fact, the early-'80s are rife with incipient disability consciousness. Think tanks such as Ed Roberts' World Institute on Disability, in Oakland, are launched. The UN, not satisfied with the success of its International Year of Disabled Persons, dubs 1983 to 1992 the International Decade of Disabled Persons. At the same time, telephones for people with hearing impairments (TTYs and TDDs) become legally required in many public places. Sears becomes the first big retailer to sell decoders for closed captioning on TV, now a required technology in every television. Even Wheaties gets in on the act; in 1984, it features a wheelchair racer on its cereal boxes!

***

Perhaps if I'd been more in touch with this wave—if I'd believed it was going to build and last—I wouldn't have been so miserable at Harvard. On the other hand, my ballooning, suffocating sense of isolation had other, more immediate causes as well.

A month after Mom died, Dad began urging Alec and me to sell the apartment we'd just inherited—our childhood home on Central Park West.

"Why do two boys in college need a six-room apartment at one of New York's premier addresses?" he asked. Well, growled. "The maintenance is a thousand a month, and it needs a lot more than that to keep it from falling apart!"

This weighs on me. Dad's wincing at the financial squeeze of having two sons at Harvard, plus my attendants, is reasonable and understandable . . . and yet, to Alec and me, this land grab rings as disingenuous and underhanded. Mom, who grew up in poverty, never trusted Dad about money. We remember their divorce-era haggling. We've known Dad to plead poverty—to complain when the price of a bagel went up to a quarter!—and yet not cut back on vacations, restaurants, or theater tickets.

Besides, Mom told us it would be ours. If she survived, she said, she would marry Bob and live with him. The Beresford apartment would be ours.

But it wasn't hers to give. Though he moved out nearly a decade ago, Dad still owned half. In fact, under the laws of joint ownership, he could now claim the whole property for himself! He only wants his half, though—and he wants us to sell ours.

It gets ugly. Lawyers become involved. We hold him off for two years. The summer after my junior year the apartment will finally be sold.

And Dad and Barbara will promptly go out and buy a vacation home on Nantucket.

***

Dad also seeks financial aid from the government. For a time, I receive marginal assistance from Connecticut's vocational rehabilitation department, an agency set up to fund needed equipment and services to get disabled people gainfully employed. It's difficult, however, to justify a liberal-arts education (especially an out-of-state one) as vocationally practical, so that coffer soon runs dry.

And I begin receiving SSI—the federal Supplemental Security Income program enacted nine years earlier, in 1972, for the indigent disabled and elderly. I temporarily collect about three hundred bucks a month.

In the news, Reagan is still attempting to gut both Section 504 of the Rehabilitation Act of 1973, which is the basis of my claim on accessibility at Harvard, and the Education for All Handicapped Children Act of 1975. Disability activists and others manage to generate an estimated forty-thousand opposition letters; in time the Administration relents.

So Reagan next cracks down on federal-benefits "abusers." It's part of a political trade-off. Congress is upending employment *dis*incentives embedded in many assistance programs, enabling folks to work part-time while continuing to receive partial benefits. At the same time, a bunch of other needy people are summarily cut off. There are reports of suicides as a result.

I'm well into my sophomore year when I receive a letter canceling my SSI and summoning me to my local Social Security office. The drab low-rise building where the Harvard van service (there are two vehicles now; I had to beg to be taken off-campus) delivers me feels, from the inside, almost hermetically sealed. By and by, the pleasant crew-cutted man who welcomes me—who might in later years have been the model for Dilbert—informs me matter-of-factly that I no longer qualify for SSI and probably never did. I'm not poor enough for benefits. Plus I have to pay back what I've already received!

I'm in no serious danger from this, but I don't want to be a patsy either. Still, there's nothing I can do. I'm one of thousands—perhaps hundreds of thousands—to fall on Reagan's chopping block.

Oddly enough, I'm almost simultaneously notified I'll soon be receiving something called Social Security Disability Insurance Survivors Benefits, which are drawn on Mom's Social Security account. Again, about three-hundred dollars a month. Welcome to the vertiginous merry-go-round of government-sponsored confusion!

In all, it's a zero-sum gain. The amount I owe SSI is deducted incrementally from my new SSDISB payments.

***

Then comes the curious case of Baby Doe—a Bloomington, Indiana, infant born with Down syndrome *and* a blocked esophagus. Surgeons say they can fix the esophagus, but the parents refuse because, as *Time* magazine reports in 1983, "nothing could be done to prevent retardation." (This is around the time Garbage Pail Kids become a popular and much-maligned toy.)

In the end, Baby Doe is sadly allowed to starve to death. "The parents' right to this choice was twice challenged in the courts by the hospital and twice upheld," the *Time* article continues. But public outcry will grow so great that in 1984 Reagan will sign the Baby Doe Law to protect disabled newborns.

I, oblivious, get Baby Doe mixed up with Baby Doc, the soon-to-be-deposed president of Haiti.

The Baby Doe incident breeds a strange symbiosis between progressive disability-rights activists and reactionary conservative types. In time, both camps will oppose using prenatal screening—for Down syndrome and other genetic "defects" (like mine)—to justify selective abortions. Later still, when Jack Kevorkian offers folks with multiple sclerosis an easy way out, the disparate viewpoints will again sound as one.

If I pay any attention at all, I'm left confused. My tendency is to try to understand all sides. I see myself as a bridge maker, not an advocate. I will come to grasp the idea that, for many disability-rights activists, these issues have nothing to do with the Sanctity of Life in a religious sense. Rather, what's at stake for them is equal protection under the law for folks deemed hopeless or useless or terminal, simply because of disabling conditions and other "abnormalities."

***

Feeling unmoored, lost at sea, I grow increasingly but secretly despondent. I lean on my reputation as a cheerful optimist like on a crutch, though this smacks more and more of wishful thinking, a desire to return to the security of the past.

Harvard is a bad place to be sad. There's little comfort to be squeezed from its cold, hard, ancient bricks and hyper-competitive population. Making matters worse—sealing my fate of loneliness— is the administration's maddening breach of promise.

At the end of freshman year, I'd learned I still could not have regular roommates even upon moving into the upper-class Houses. The Deans had thought they could accommodate my urgent request, even encouraging me to choose from among a short list of options—primarily, a small rooming group in Currier House, off the old Radcliffe quad (roughly equivalent to campus Siberia), or a big suite in Mather House usually reserved for seniors. I toured both and chose Mather. Then the Deans reneged.

They alleged Mather hadn't been tested for safe, adequate accessibility. (Not that Quincy House, where they ultimately dumped me, was exactly up to code.) Second—reminiscent of the previous year's excuse—my taking a senior suite as a sophomore just wouldn't be fair to the other students.

In retrospect, it was blatant segregation (separate *isn't* equal)! But I didn't raise much of a fuss. I didn't want to be unreasonable. Becoming accessible was a total transmogrification for Harvard's hoary old campus.

The *Harvard Crimson* got wind of the story:

> His commitment to living a full, normal life led Mattlin to
> select Mather as his housing choice this spring, . . . primarily
> because it has only large suites, where he would have

roommates—potential "buddies" who could relieve some of the "great strain" of living only with an attendant on whom he relies heavily.

. . . Although Mattlin will reluctantly take his belongings to a House with limited wheelchair accessibility and no suites for the disabled, he will undoubtedly arrive at Quincy . . . with the same outgoing attitude and distinct sense of humor that helped him through high school and his freshman year at Harvard. "It'll be a really tight squeeze," Mattlin says of the wheelchair route to the Quincy House dining hall. "There's the smell of garbage, and you have to go through the kitchen," he adds, accurately but humorously.

Alas, even this publicity is to no avail.

I move into the very same drab two-room unit previously occupied by the only other wheelchair-using undergrad in recent memory. I briefly contemplate hanging a sign on the door that reads: Handicapped Unit.

Yet I do my best to fit in at Quincy House. I like its un-snobbish, unintimidating reputation as a place to party. I become a regular at the in-house Q-World Grill. I'm a fan of its uniquely Bostonian (at least to me) vertically split hotdogs and "frappes." A hand-scrawled sign above the counter reads, "If you don't see it on the menu, ask for it." Translation: Beer. Since Massachusetts raised the drinking age to twenty-one, this is supposedly the only way it can be sold. I happily indulge.

I have a new attendant—a tall soft-spoken man named Clayton, whom Dad found through a classified ad in the *Times*, or somewhere. Later, I'll find out that while I'm at the Grill, Clayton is calling Dad and telling him I'm crying every night, which is untrue. Dad offers to drive up, but Clayton tells him he's taking care of it.

At the same time, I have a new weekend guy named Seamus. Seamus is formerly of the Irish merchant marines, complete with a heavy brogue. He hand rolls his own tobacco cigarettes while telling tall tales of his travels. (I realize this sounds like a stereotype, but it's true!) A crowd gathers around him at the Quincy dining hall. One of my classmates even follows us back to the Handicapped Unit after dinner to hear more.

On his second or third Sunday, Seamus tells me in confidence that Clayton made a pass at him. It's awkward, the two of them sharing a small bedroom every weekend. I had thought Clayton would return to Oneonta, his hometown, on weekends, but that isn't happening.

"Are you serious?" I ask. Implication: Or is this more of your blarney?

"Aye! An' ah'm quittin' if this kinda thing is alloo'ed to g' on!"

On Monday, after Seamus has left, I talk to Clayton. Delicately.

"Did anything go on this weekend between you and Seamus?"

"No. Not really. But I think he's gay."

Clayton's version is that Seamus was the one doing the nocturnal nudging.

I know I must act decisively, before the next weekend. On Wednesday, I resolve to be loyal to my weekday help. He's the one who's really depending on this job. So I call a few of my second-choice candidates for the weekend position— the ones I'd turned down for Seamus just a few weeks earlier. Jay, still interested, is hired on the spot. That settled, I call Seamus to say it's not working out.

I needn't have bothered. On Friday afternoon Clayton disappears. The Harvard van drops me at Quincy after class (I've been going around without an attendant as much as possible), and when I return to the Handicapped Unit he's cleared out.

What to do? I don't have a good back-up plan, but I have kept Bill's phone number from last year. Miraculously, he's able to start on Monday (till then I'll have Jay). Plus he has family in the area to visit on weekends.

I never see Clayton again, but he does leave me with one remembrance. A few weeks later I receive a phone bill for eight hundred dollars! (It's two months' worth. I presume he removed the previous month's bill when he brought up my mail, and I never noticed.)

I call Clayton's former home in Oneonta, to where I'm guessing he's returned. "Oh my God!" says his ex-roommate, when I deliver my news. "You too? Hey, you're lucky—that bastard still owes *me* a grand!"

***

Buffeted by revolving attendants, intractable Harvard deans, the loss of Mom, and the imminent forfeiture of my childhood home, is it any wonder that, at nineteen, I have the panicky sensation of losing my grip on the only anchors left?

I grow thin from lack of eating and have no patience for schoolwork. I fall asleep in class and study only sporadically (in fairness, that could have something to do with Max Weber and John Locke). I like writing term papers but despise research. When I say research, I'm referring to *book* research. I don't do lab experiments or interview expert sources—and there is no Internet yet.

Book research poses two problems, neither of which I'm yet equipped to recognize. The first has to do with libraries. I enter Lamont Library by ramp (the larger Widener Library requires a more circuitous entrance) and attempt to direct my attendant to finger through the card catalog. I can't actually peer into the small drawers myself—except for the few that happen to be at my exact height. So there's a lot of whispering back and forth, and I have to trust my attendant's comprehension skills.

(Eventually I will learn to ask the reference librarian, which speeds things up tremendously. It forces me to explain myself better than I can to my attendants, plus the librarians frequently contribute their own valuable insights. Good old-fashioned service is often the best accessibility accommodation!)

Once I have the books I need, it's incredibly difficult manipulating them. I concede that I'm a "bad reader," plodding slowly through dense prose, easily becoming bored. But in truth I'm struggling as much with the logistics—angling the texts to reduce glare, turning pages, cross-referencing to other books and other passages in the same book, highlighting, Post-It noting, and simultaneous note-taking—all things I can't do.

To be sure, that's what the attendant is for. But attendants are not scholars, generally speaking. And even to this day I feel there is a bubble that forms—or *should* form—around you and the material you're working to master. So having to direct each step of the process verbally—that is, to instruct my hired help how to help—can be more than an interruption; it can be an intrusion.

Perhaps this is an excuse, I fear in my college years. Perhaps I'm simply a lazy student. All I can say for sure is the process of information gathering and fact checking is prohibitively exhausting in those pre-computer days.

I fare better in psychology and literature classes, fortunately, where I feel greater liberty to offer freewheeling interpretations. I'm heartened by the rumor that the hardest part about Harvard is getting in, not staying in. Not that I'm anywhere near failing; it just feels like I am.

***

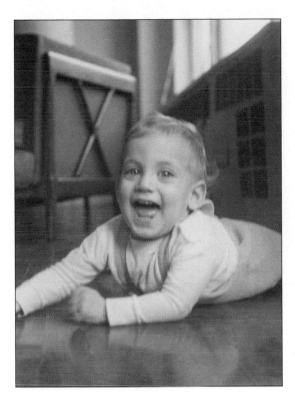

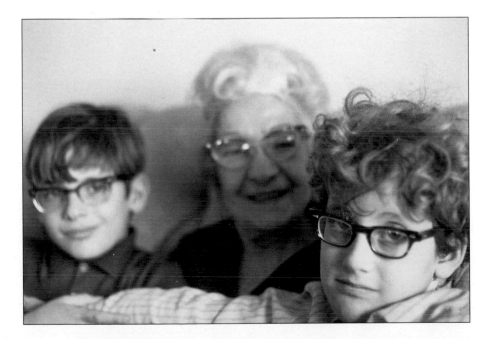

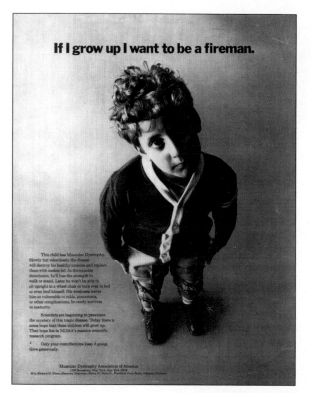

If I grow up I want to be a fireman.

This child has Muscular Dystrophy.
Slowly but relentlessly the disease
will destroy his healthy muscles and replace
them with useless fat. As the muscles
deteriorate, he'll lose the strength to
walk or stand. Later he won't be able to
sit upright in a wheel chair or turn over in bed
or even feed himself. His weakness leaves
him so vulnerable to colds, pneumonia,
or other complications, he rarely survives
to maturity.

Scientists are beginning to penetrate
the mystery of this tragic disease. Today there is
some hope that these children will grow up.
That hope lies in MDAA's massive scientific
research program.

Only your contributions keep it going.
Give generously.

Muscular Dystrophy Association of America
1790 Broadway, New York, New York 10019
Mrs. Richard M. Nixon, Honorary Chairman; Henry M. Watts Jr., President Jerry Lewis, National Chairman

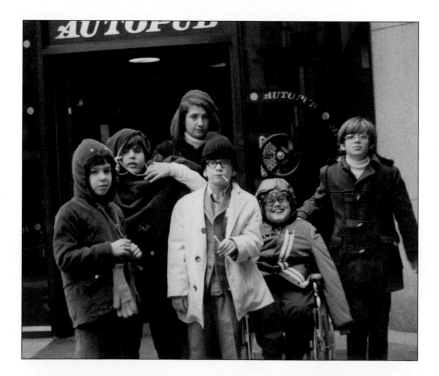

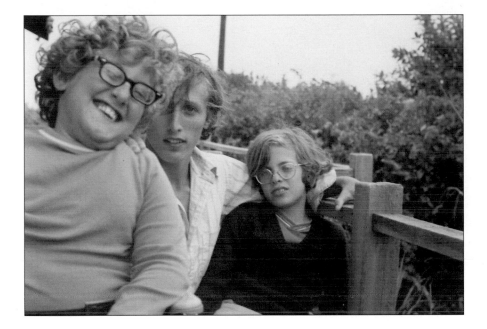

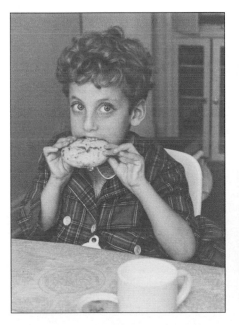

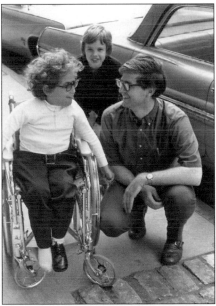

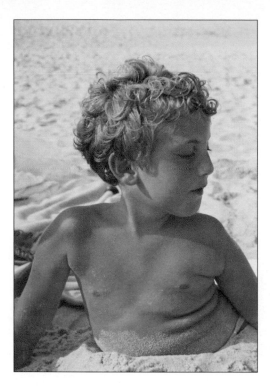

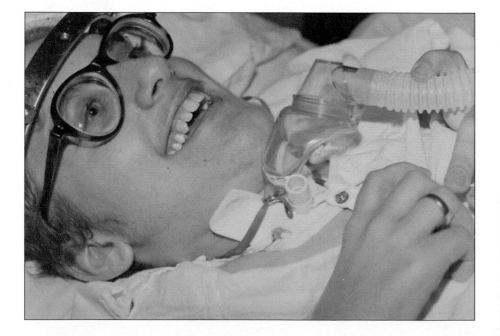

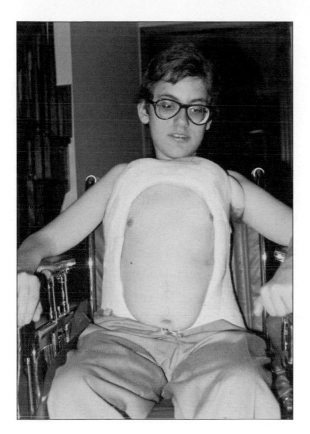

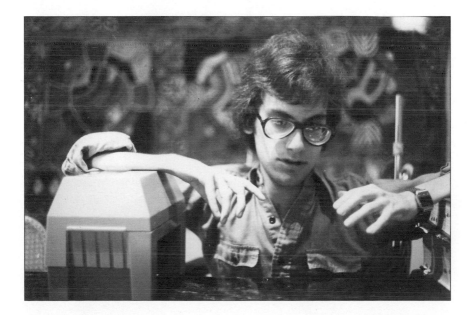

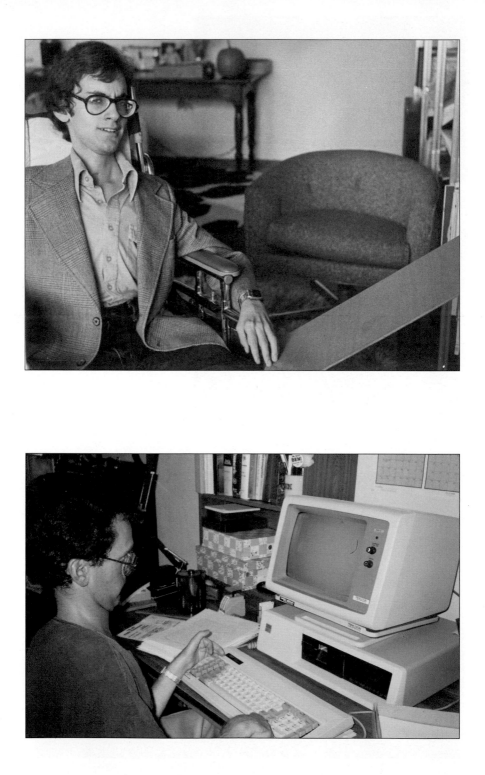

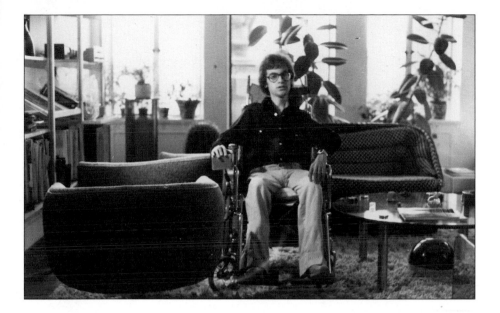

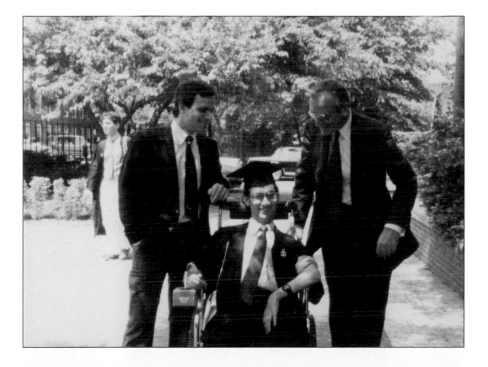

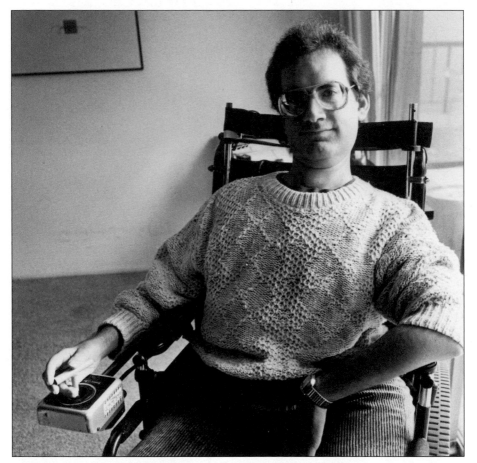
Photo by Theodora Litsios. As first appeared in the March 1993 issue of *SELF* magazine.

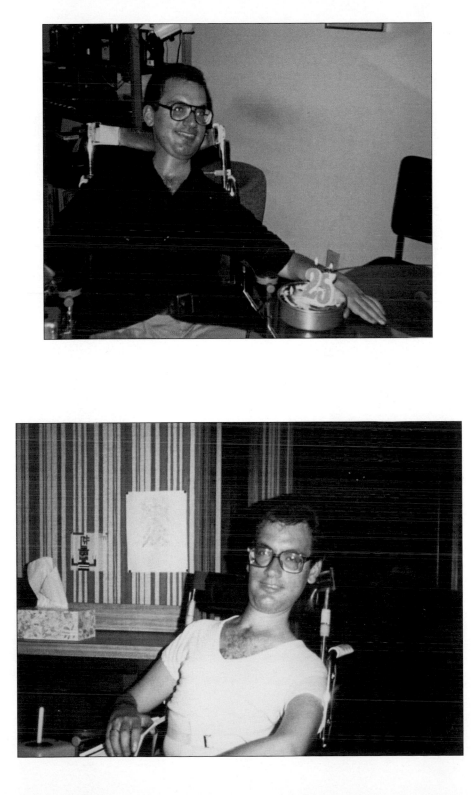

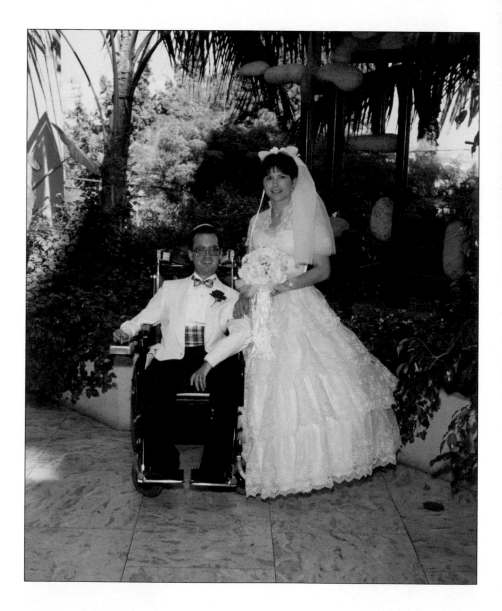

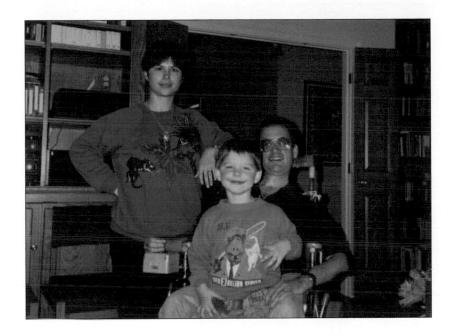

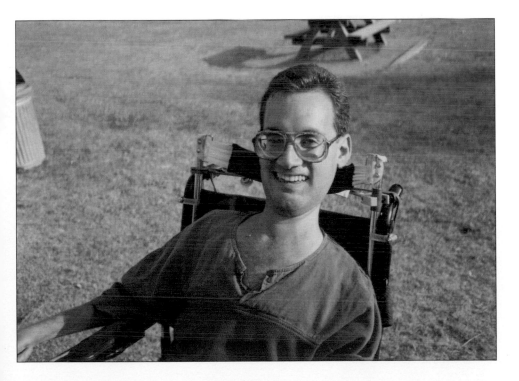

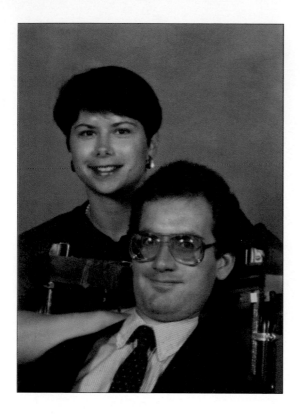

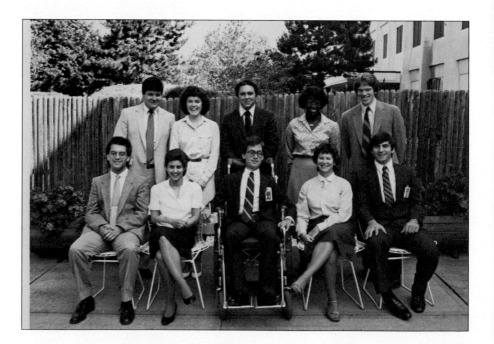

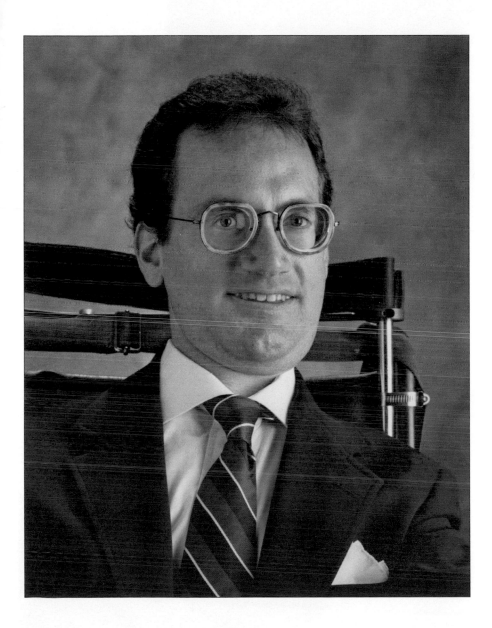

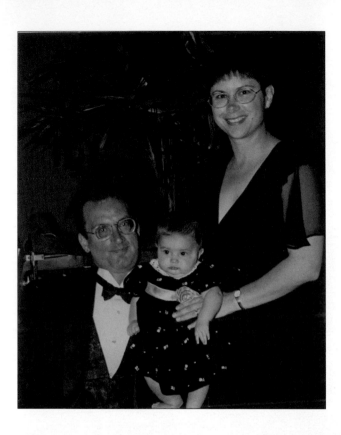

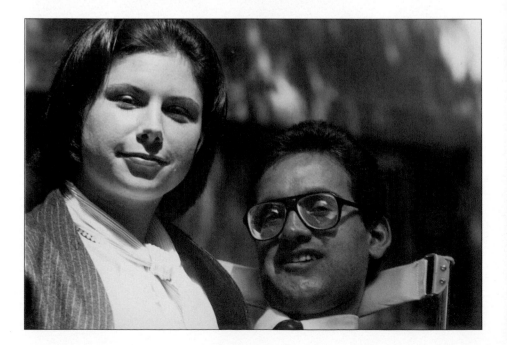

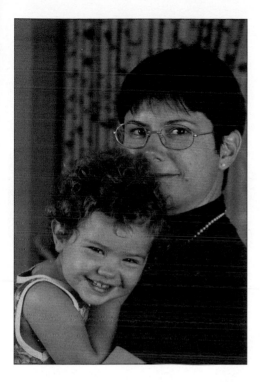

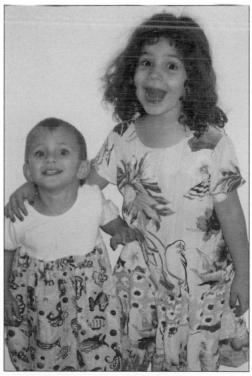

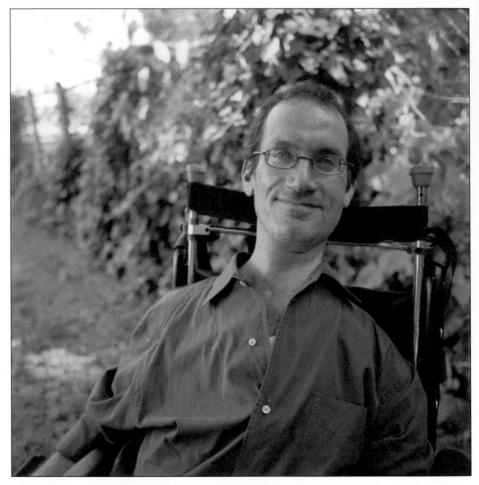

Photo by Danny Rothenberg/Polaris for *Newsweek*. As first appeared in the July 24, 2006, issue of *Newsweek*.

Alfred Lord Tennyson famously observed that, in the spring, a young man's fancy turns to thoughts of love. It's not only in the spring.

I'm overwhelmed at Harvard. I crave ballast. And at nineteen, the ego boost I seek is a girlfriend. So I ask out a series of female friends; shyness is not my problem. Every one accepts. We have dinner—I never eat much at those dinners, of course, because it's too awkward to feed myself—or attend a concert or movie . . . and we talk and laugh, maybe even hold hands . . . but never kiss, except possibly a peck on the cheek.

With each encounter I'm plumbing for a profound connection, a revelation about my destiny. To me, women hold eternal and transcendental secrets—they must!—and I'm desperate to fashion a key and glimpse inside. Such sharing might come in time, but I'm in accelerated mode—scrounging for Depth (with a capital D) with greater intensity and celerity than any modern concept of "speed dating" or online compatibility testing would dare attempt. I recall Christine, Myra, Jennifer, Caroline, Beth, and many others.

It's after midnight when I bid one of them good night with a frank if flowery confession: "I would ask you for a kiss before parting, which I had intended and practiced, but it's too soon, I realize now. It's only a few months since my mother died, you see, and I don't dare even contemplate a real, lasting relationship with anyone. I'm so sorry."

Do I really say such words, or only imagine them? Not that the poor young lady implies any interest in pursuing things further. It's cold out, her hands buried in her coat pockets, and odds are she just wants to go home. I strain to accept her abrupt back-step, the way her eyes pop wide. "That's cool," she says. "Really."

"You understand, then?"

"No problem, Ben. Good night now."

In my still-new motorized wheelchair, I make my way back to Quincy House trembling against the biting chill wind. I hadn't the courage to ask my date to help me don my coat or gloves, and have left my attendant back in the dorm for privacy's sake. My fingers stiffen on the chair's control stick, and I wonder intermittently if I'll make it back at all.

I do. I always do. I never learn to ask a passing stranger for help, nor to set up a time at which the attendant should come looking for me. (If only we'd had cell phones then!)

More humiliating still is the junior I fall for as a sophomore. By my calculus, if women are linked to an essential, fundamental truth, older women must be even more so. They wield a greater command over how things ought to be, and so offer greater comfort.

My beguiling inamorata is in an "open relationship" with another guy—a senior! I play it cool at first, or try to. Until one night I'm waiting in Quincy House for her call . . . her roommate, who answers when I break down and call, says she's gone out. I wait some more. I'm certain I've seen a look in her eyes that implies interest. A magnetic echo-signal that says *soul mate*. As I wait, I have Bill turn on my old black-and-white portable TV. I reluctantly find myself glued to *It Happened One Night*. I watch Clark Gable take charge of amatory chaos, ordering Claudette Colbert (and everyone else) around with such manly charm that the effect is magical. When at long last my phone does ring, I berate and cajole my fantasy girl (à la Clark Gable) into meeting at the Kong. Which is the Hong Kong, a Chinese restaurant famous for its lounge scene and easy carding policy. Bill walks me over and, when my date shows up, he dutifully vanishes. We share a ground-floor booth (the real action, I'm told, is upstairs but there's no elevator) and a Dragon Bowl—a large vessel of a rum-based concoction.

My date, though older, gets asked for ID; as usual I do not.

The dark, smoky place is crowded and loud. We shout and laugh at what we think the other one is saying. I warm up from within and begin feeling good when all of a sudden my date's attention is snatched away. "Look!" she says by way of explanation. "There's John!"

John is her "real" boyfriend, or in my interpretation my chief rival for her affections. I know John, through my brother. Nice enough, but I'm sure he doesn't see in her what I see. He lands about two tables down from us, with a group. Frankly, he seems indifferent to us, but she keeps smiling and waving at him. I hasten us out as speedily as possible.

Back on Mass Ave I perceive how drunk I am. A passerby makes a joke about being careful not to lose my chair-driving license. I've heard the joke before but guffaw politely. My date and I amble back to Quincy House, and it's only gradually that I get the sense she's concerned I might not get there safely without her.

She does not even enter my rooms. She announces she's going back to her place, which is on the other side of campus. Not taking the hint, I insist on accompanying her. To make sure I'm able to return safely afterward, I suggest Bill tag along. It *is* a long walk, after all. He follows from a polite distance.

The next morning when I wake up with a pounding headache, Bill asks if I remember shouting "I love you! I love you! I love you!" across Kirkland Street. I dimly recall telling her she'd better break up with John because I needed a serious commitment, but refute actually saying the L word.

Needless to say, I've never spoken with the young woman since. Not even on Facebook.

***

That summer—one year after Mom's death—something within me sharpens. I'll no longer search for true love, I decide. I'm going to focus on the single goal of losing my virginity. After all, I'll be twenty in a few months!

Doubtless it's a stand-in for happiness, a shortcut to improving self-esteem, but...

I don't *feel* like a virgin. And in my mind I'm not. I have no soft-focus illusions about the act, no expectation of doves flying or firecrackers sounding. I've read enough Updike to know the moist, sticky, smelly slog of it. And I'm sufficiently self-aware to realize I'm not exactly anybody's idea of a stud, though I envisage myself to be a pretty smooth operator.

In June, back in New York, I meet with my old pal Jane from high school. She's the one who predicted I'd go to Harvard and write for the *New Yorker*. She's home from college, too, but don't ask me which one.

It's one of those disgustingly humid evenings when everyone looks frazzled and "glowing." But to me, she looks good enough. She's interested in literature—and more importantly, in *my* literature. I tell her about my short story but complain it's not as good as Updike. I expect her to say, Who is? Instead, she offers this: "You don't need to be as good as Updike. You need to be as good as Ben Mattlin. To write as well as *you* can."

I could have fallen in love with her for this wisdom, but I'm no longer looking for love.

We "walk" from a café back to my place, a short distance. It's one of my final stays at the Beresford. She reclines on my sofa and I put it to her: "Can I kiss you?"

I've never understood what's meant by a "sideways glance" until that moment.

"No," she comes back quickly. "We're good friends, yes, but I've never thought of you *that* way."

I've never thought of you that way becomes a running theme with the women I target. Later, I'll gather it's a common theme for many with disabilities. We're safe enough and patient enough to confide in—confide in deeply—but we're basically considered sexless. Disqualified before we try. Out of the running, so to speak.

So I scratch Jane off my mental list and go on undeterred.

Persistence is a family trait. I grew up hearing, *Don't take no for an answer* (this, of course, presumes you are not a latent rapist!) and *What have you got to lose by trying?* Mom, post-divorce, scrounged for forever to get back into the workforce. Dad, even now, in his eighties, sends out manuscripts and queries with ruthless efficiency as he tries—with some success—to place his wry, bittersweet essays about aging.

But I suspect I would've been a stubborn cuss anyway, just by virtue of having to be—in order to survive. For me, sometimes the very act of breathing itself is a game of wills.

By August I'm spending a lot of time in Stamford, at Dad and Barbara's. I left an internship in the city, at a famous rehab clinic on the East Side, when I realized it was one of those do-goodery keep-a-cripple-busy programs. I should've been clued in when the woman who interviewed me asked where I was in school and then said, "Harvard? Where's that?"

"Cambridge, Massachusetts. Near Boston. You know, Harvard University—"

She nearly fell over backwards. "Oh, *that* Harvard! Hmmm—"

Not to knock the value of these occupational-rehab programs. Young men and women with all manner (and combinations) of disabilities, few educational or professional prospects, and even less in the way of financial resources, learn to answer telephones and direct calls or dish out cafeteria trays and other essential skills, earn a few bucks and feel good about themselves. But after two weeks I was certain I didn't belong. Ostensibly, I was helping put together a newsletter for participants. But there was no adaptive technology available to help me figure out how to become more employable. I was just marking time, filling a space. Besides, there were at least three guys in the program named Rocko! It was a different world.

At Dad and Barbara's, I soak up rays shirtless in their front yard and listen to WNEW. I'd developed a bad rash on my back anyway, which needed time to air, I reasoned. A few days of this and I grow restless. My half-brother

Jeff is now five and off at day camp all day. His summertime nanny is a recent college grad from California.

No, she's not blonde and leggy and doesn't sashay around in a bikini. Her dark brown hair is cut short, and she wears glasses over her wide brown eyes. She's come every summer for the past two years, so we're used to each other. Most importantly, she's used to *me*—the way I eat, the way I get lifted into and out of the Checker car, the way I rely on Dad or other help to get up in the morning and to bed at night, and the way I look with no shirt on.

I'd never paid her much mind before, other than noticing her large chest. But this summer she's developed a delightful insouciance—doesn't fly off the handle with rash, pretentious opinions as I'd at least imagined she did on our previous encounters. She's more sure of herself, or rather more comfortable in her own skin, notwithstanding the occasional self-effacing giggle. Her wide-ranging intelligence and creative competence are evident in the way she challenges Jeff's mind—telling stories with plenty of questions for him to ponder—whips up inventive art projects and challenging recipes in the kitchen (all part of her nanny duties), and in the evenings—after sharing a bottle of wine with Barbara—quotes Keats, Milton, and PG Wodehouse all while cracking shockingly naughty jokes.

MaryLois is my logical next victim.

***

After dinner one night, I suggest we take a walk. She agrees. In a clearing, she sits on a low stone wall while we chat. I tell her about things I like to do in New York. She tells me about her graduate school plans. We agree that Stamford is tiresome.

By moving my motorized wheelchair in close, I'm able to walk my left hand onto her blue-jeaned right thigh. She doesn't push it off. Mentally, I search through my store of role models from TV and movies. Clark Gable might just grab her and plant a kiss. Not an option for me. For me, it has to be verbal. I have to get her participation, her complicity. But how?

Captain Kirk. There's an episode of *Star Trek* that ends with him kissing a blonde (okay, there are dozens of those) on the *Enterprise* bridge. First he says something about having to remain in command; then she asks if a kiss would pose too great a disruption.

MaryLois is a bit in the Captain Kirk role, it occurs to me. She has far-ranging responsibilities as a nanny and feels she must maintain a degree of decorum. Plus, she admits, she likes to be right, in control.

So I say, "Would it cause too much of a disturbance if I were to ask for a kiss?"

Later, she'll tell me she was tempted to slap my face and walk away, but decided a better way to knock my smirk off was to go ahead and kiss me—hard, voraciously—then declare it's time to go home.

I arrange to meet her later that night, after Dad has gotten me ready for bed and gone to bed himself. Or maybe I just decide that on my own.

Near midnight, I'm in my room, in pajamas, waiting for her. She doesn't come, so I wheel down the hall to her room, tap the door ajar with my footrest, and softly say, "Knock knock" (because I can't actually raise my arm to do it).

She sits in bed in her white and pink cotton nightgown and I park my chair beside. She has a small TV and we watch—honest!—a *Star Trek* rerun. After a while, I suggest we pick up where we left off outside. It's always verbal with me.

After we've kissed a while, I urge her to undress. She shakes her head. "You'll have to do that yourself," she says.

"I would if I could."

"Not tonight, it won't happen. I have to get Jeff to camp in the morning."

Regardless, I deliver the spiel I've worked out in my head. "You should know that I have weak muscles but full sensation. Everything works. I can't climb on top, but don't worry about hurting me. I'm not delicate. And it's not contagious."

She nods but doesn't budge. Before I leave her room—before I go down the hall and wake Dad to lift me into bed—she kisses me on the top of the head. Disappointed, I nevertheless take this as encouragement.

A few days later she meets me at my apartment in the city—in its final days; we agree to go to a free outdoor Elvis Costello concert. Buses and taxis aren't yet wheelchair accessible, so we "walk" the thirty blocks to the West Side pier. She's in heels and a slinky pink cocktail dress, and men on the streets whistle and growl. On the return trek, I offer to ride her on my lap but she refuses. We stop for a drink. I buy her a flower. Though my intentions are carnal, I know my only chance of winning her is with cornball romance.

Back at the apartment—glad it's still mine, for a little while longer at least—I ask if she'd prefer to sleep alone. I'm trying to be polite, but she almost seems insulted. I let her know I'm happy that she expects us to sleep together. I suggest she change in Mom's old bathroom and not come out till I call.

My temporary attendant changes me in the other room and then politely sets me down in Mom's old king-size bed. Once he's left the room, I tell her the coast is clear.

More overnight dates follow. At the end of the summer we decide we don't want this to end. I don't know exactly what she sees in me, but I believe she's eager to escape her small-town upbringing. In addition, she's at a bit of a loose end work- and school-wise. I imagine she needs a calling, a sense of direction. Perhaps my complex life feels to her like something akin to a force of nature.

What she tells me is that, as a woman of just five-foot-two, she feels safe knowing I won't dominate or hurt her physically. So ML stays on at Dad and Barbara's and visits me in Cambridge every weekend. By the following June, though the Beresford is sold, I propose we live together. I am twenty.

Having aced the GRE but failed to get into a graduate program she likes, ML is amenable to just about anything. And I can't take any more wrenching Sunday night departures. Every time, I cry uncontrollable torrents—only dimly aware that I've been saving up tears for nearly two years. Ever since Mom died.

CHAPTER EIGHT

IF NO ONE NOTICES A DISABILITY, DOES IT REALLY EXIST?

1984-1990

"For me, everything's too much and nothing's enough."
—Mary Karr, *Lit: A Memoir*

Somewhere in Oklahoma, it's raining big, loud drops on the echoey raised roof of my shit-brown Ford Econoline 150 cargo van. The van, which I'd bought near Boston with Mom's life insurance money, isn't pretty but it does the job. That is, it's big enough to fit me in my motorized wheelchair, and pretty much all my worldly possessions. *Our* worldly possessions, I should say.

ML—who's driving—and I are en route to Los Angeles. Her family is there. We're switching coasts, switching family-roots, welding a new life together.

On the van's intermittent radio we hear about Ronald Reagan's reelection. The first presidential race in which I'm old enough to vote, and it's a disappointment. We'd both cast absentee ballots for Mondale, back in Connecticut before our big departure. Somehow being a college-graduate-slash-adult means registering as a Democrat.

(The election also happens to be the first under a new Voting Accessibility for the Elderly and Handicapped law, the provisions of which I innocently circumvent by voting absentee.)

Our new life includes a wheelchair lift on the van, thanks to Connecticut's fickle vocational rehab department, which had evaluated me as unable to drive, even with hand controls. That's okay. A born and bred New Yorker, I don't exactly yearn to take the wheel.

In my wheelchair, I'm strapped in behind the driver's seat. We've attached a tray table to my chair to hold snacks and a book. I try reading aloud to help ML stay awake and keep us connected, but the monster van has terrible acoustics and I'm not loud enough.

It takes five days to reach her childhood home—during which she's my only attendant. This in itself is a bold development, a turning point. I'd been resisting having her do anything custodial for me, but the payoff in privacy—from parents and from paid outsiders—tips the scales. Plus ML really wanted to. She wanted to contribute to my well-being.

During my senior year at Harvard—while she earned a master's in education and a teaching credential—we'd shared a two-bedroom apartment in Cambridge. Bill occupied the second bedroom on weeknights, Jay on weekends. So other than occasionally turning me at night in the bed we shared, ML did none of my caretaking. (Even at that, I tried not to wake her too often.)

The problem was, the paid attendants never took as good care of me as she could. Over time she wore me down with small kindnesses that grew bigger, more personal. Such as re-shaving my sideburns to even them out. Or plucking my most egregious nose hairs. Years later I'd become suspicious, even resentful, of how, for her—to steal an apt phrase I'd glom on to from an article about someone else—the validation of serving others could become a substitute for self-directed wisdom. But at the time I came to like, then depend on, her attentions.

One day, we drove in her car to visit a friend. When it was time to go home, there was no one to help lift me back into the car. So ML tried it herself. The discovery that she could lift me was revelatory! For a woman of five-foot-two, she has surprising upper-body strength!

Accelerating our itch to fly free was the odd way Bill had grown resentful . . . territorial as a mountain lion. "Now that you're sharing a bigger bed," he'd announced shortly after we moved to the sunny, thin-walled Cambridge apartment, "let's say we alternate days making the bed, hmm? I'll do Monday-Wednesday-Friday, and you, MaryLois, can take Tuesdays and Thursdays—type thing."

Yet soon she lost track of the schedule she hadn't ever really agreed to in the first place. So Bill unilaterally took to making *half* the bed each morning. (I kid you not!) I wonder now how miffed he must've been to discover neither she nor I cared much whether or how the bed was made. Most days it stayed just as he left it, half-made.

ML's haphazard housekeeping wasn't Bill's only target. He'd complain about Jay after the weekend shift—the way he'd parked my commode chair (a bare-bones wheelchair with a hole in the seat, which rolls over the toilet), for example. "It should be *here*, not there," he'd holler, though no one but myself was around. "Tell him to cut it out!"

Bill's idiosyncratic tantrums aside, I was learning a key skill: How to juggle multiple attendants—maximizing each one's strengths, trading off tasks, constructing flexible boundaries, soothing egos.

Still, Bill was becoming scary. Yet the more prickly he became, the more snugly ML and I bonded. More and more it felt like us against the world.

After graduation, there wasn't much keeping us in the Northeast Corridor. We spent the summer in Connecticut, at Dad and Barbara's (with a new part-time helper, who didn't last long). ML completed leftover course work and I found a temporary job at IBM. I wrote short articles for employee newsletters—one of a team of student interns at a corporation eager to flaunt its progressive hiring policies. Suit and tie every day. Somehow managed to feed myself small cheese sandwiches at lunch, with minimal help from coworkers. Hand-wrote my articles (there were plenty of secretaries to type them). Mostly I watched the clock.

That was the summer of IBM's ubiquitous ads introducing the PC as a device so simple even Charlie Chaplin's tramp could use it. Only I couldn't. At least not for a few years.

Knowing the internship would end in September, I took a lot of time off to interview at magazine and book publishers in New York. But even graduating cum laude from Harvard didn't guarantee a young man in a wheelchair so much as an entry-level proofreading job!

Alec had moved to Philadelphia, where he was building a career in survey research. And the bubbling-acid rift between Dad and me—ignited over his nagging need to sell my childhood apartment—was smoldering still. So when ML learned LA was desperately hiring teachers, we had no excuse not to go.

***

It's a warm November evening, around sunset, when we arrive at her family's comfortable ranch-style house in a Los Angeles suburb. Nervous energy fills the air. After a sumptuous dinner of home-smoked turkey, homemade egg bread, and I forget what else—filled with questions and answers and nostalgia—her mother vanishes and then reappears in the living room . . . dressed like a sprite or wood nymph, or maybe Robin Hood: Green tights, blousy beige top with a cinch neck, and cockeyed black cap.

"Well?" she asks.

A hearty round of approval from all. ML's younger sister is there. Her two older siblings have moved out. I smile and try not to act confused.

It turns out ML's mom is off to a dress rehearsal at a local theater. I never do learn the name of the show.

In random discussions and over nonstop eating—the kitchen *is* the family center—it's evident they're smart and creative and loving and just the right amount of kooky. Much less formal than most families I've known. But what they make of me remains to be seen. (I wonder now how I'd feel if my daughter brought home a quadriplegic paramour. Wouldn't I worry whether she knew what she was getting into?)

Like Woody Allen in that scene in *Annie Hall* where, facing Diane Keaton's WASP family, he imagines he's turned into a Hasidic Jew in full black-hatted garb and *peyos*, I become acutely self-conscious. They're rugged Westerners, ML's clan. Not roughnecks but do-it-yourselfers. Which frankly seems exotic next to my background, yet rattles me because it's so suffused with basic, hands-on physicality.

After a few days, as they're helping us move to an apartment we've found—particularly when her hardy, robust dad, a noted engineer and research physicist, and visiting older brother, an intimidatingly handsome aspiring screenwriter, are hauling a sofa we'd purchased—I'm painfully aware for the first time in my life of being a true cripple.

"I feel so damn useless," I hear myself mutter.

***

Unbeknownst to us, the small apartment we've found is in what will become the notorious Rampart District (see the Denzel Washington movie *Training Day*). Our new building is actually a converted hotel built in the 1940s; we love its frowsy Art Deco vibe. It's not entirely wheelchair accessible—I have to enter and exit the building via a steep ramp off the basement, because the front lobby has steps—but the price is right and we're too young (read *foolish*) to care.

After Bill's peevishness, we've decided against having another live-in attendant, so it's just a one-bedroom. I'll find someone for daytime, as I had in high school. ML will take evenings and weekends. Only later, when I'll need to increase the attendant hours, will this arrangement prove a bad precedent—forcing me to ask Dad for extra money, which will feel akin to an admission of failure.

She lands work almost immediately, never mind that it's in an overcrowded inner-city school. So I get busy dialing home-health agencies out of the phone book. Monday morning, when the agency man arrives for the first time, I'm lying nude in bed—well, in the sofa bed we're using for now. It's ML's first day at work, and she mustn't be late; I don't remember if either of us thought even once about the dangers inherent here, leaving me alone and stark naked with a stranger.

I'm prepared to take charge, to tell the man all about me and what I need. But he is chatty. A short, stocky man in jeans and a T-shirt, he has a slight Southern accent and a scraggly reddish-brown goatee to complete the redneck stereotype. He keeps telling me he used to be a medical doctor back in Tennessee but his license isn't recognized here.

"Can you imagine—from a medical doctor to *this*?" he says to drive home his disillusionment.

I try to make appropriate, responsive-but-not-encouraging noises.

"And believe me when I tell you, I don't know how many of my patients used to hit on me. They'd grope me! Truth," he says. "By the way, I'm gay."

"Let's walk down to the grocery store," I say once I'm safely dressed and in my chair. I feel desperate to get out in the open air, around witnesses. Not that anything he's revealed is intrinsically scary, though it seems too much information, under the circumstances. Rather, it's something to do with his delivery that sparks a sense in me that he's itching for a fight. The timbre of his voice maybe, or a certain squint of his eyes. Something definitely feels unstable.

Walking to the grocery store is an alien concept in LA. But with my cracker ex-doctor oddball beside me, I find one—a sort of oversized bodega down the street, on the edges of Koreatown. Inside, I get flustered—the brands are different. I can't find what I'm looking for.

That evening, ML and I go out for dinner and I can't stop shaking.

Nevertheless, dunce that I am on the cusp of twenty-two, I let the frightening attendant come again the next day and for a few days after that . . .

maybe it's me, I reason. Maybe I'm prejudiced. Maybe I need to find a way to work with him . . . because, really, what choice do I have?

On Friday, finally, I place a classified ad in the LA *Times*. Over the weekend I conduct interviews. ML meets them all—the various unskilled, curious applicants who show up—but mostly stays out of the way, her distaste for these encounters barely suppressed. They are—or can be—rare windows into another slice of life, a set of different socioeconomic backgrounds. Sometimes this is wonderful—a kind of eye-opening multiculturalism—but other times it's just awkward, grating, even incendiary. I've known it to go both ways, frankly. I wish I didn't sound so hardened about it, but that's the way it is.

It's my choice, ML declares, not hers; already she's gleaned how fragile my authority can be with newcomers, how easily I'm assumed to be the patient to take care of, instead of the one who must be listened to and pleased.

So, I hire a young man—let's call him Peter. I'm perhaps too quick to overlook Peter's spotty history. He's younger than I am and even newer to LA. His only reference is his grandmother in Denver. But I like him and I'm desperate.

Peter and I get along fine despite his constantly tuning my stereo to country music. Afternoons, after I've sent out all the résumés I can for the day, I have nothing to do and Peter and I watch old sitcom reruns on TV. It's boring yet it becomes addictive. I know I should be doing something worthwhile, but what? Every day I scrounge employment ads—publishers, editors, journalists, writers, proofreaders, etc. I network with anyone I know—from Harvard's career services office to friends of friends. I score several interviews, which go smoothly. Then, nothing.

In fairness, part of the problem is I'm not suited for entry-level work. I can't be a "copy boy," jockeying papers here and there. I can't sort mail or run after burning news stories. I can't type (enter data, interface with a terminal—whatever the current expression is) quickly enough. I know I can write well, given the opportunity, and believe I can edit others. But such brainy, specialized, nonphysical jobs are reserved for those with basic experience already under their belts.

Nevertheless, I'm gradually forced to consider whether people could be judging me harshly because I'm in a wheelchair. Not just *in a wheelchair*. Let's be honest. I'm disabled from head to toe. My spine is twisted, and I'm utterly bereft of musculature.

I hesitate to admit this. I still believe I can pass. I'm not up to accusing anyone of unfair treatment, even in the abstract. But intellectually I know that denying the possibility would be foolish.

Practical questions surge up. Do I mention my disability when I apply for a job? Does it belong on my résumé? I mean, what difference should it make? Most of the disability literature I see doesn't address such real-world conundrums (bedsores and flat-tire repairs galore, however!), but that's changing, too. Somewhere I read that it's better to take control of employment questions under your own terms. So, when scheduling interviews—on the phone beforehand, not on my résumé or in my cover letters—I start asking if there are any steps or other obstacles for which I'll need to plan ahead. But potential employers still seem taken aback when they meet me.

Not until this post-college stage have I ever felt so "handicapped" by my disability.

***

One midday the phone rings. From my new speakerphone emanates the voice of one of my career-networking contacts, who's heard of an opening at the LA *Business Journal*. The editor wants to meet right away.

I instruct Peter to lie me down, strip off my jeans, pull my gray flannels on me, and put me back in the wheelchair. I teach him how to tie my necktie, just as Dad taught me. I say I'll pay overtime if this meeting runs late.

ML has taken the van to work, but the newspaper's offices are only a few blocks away. Peter walks with me, then waits in the hallway. In the side of my chair I've had him tuck a folder with my résumé and clips from the *Harvard Independent* and IBM. Which proves a good move when Dave, the editor, asks for my writing samples.

"Here," I say. "Can you reach?"

He doesn't flinch. After a time he looks up and says, "This reminds me of, like, *Esquire* or the *New Yorker*." I know he's just saying that because I'm transplanted from New York, but I'm immensely flattered—until the ax falls. "The opening I have is in research. In our library. Don't think that'd be a good match for you."

I can't honestly disagree. Then Dave comes up with a plan.

"Do you freelance?" he asks.

A few days later, over the phone, we settle on the idea of a diary of a successful ad. To my delight, the story practically writes itself. The ad: The still-famous Super Bowl spot introducing Mac computers ("see why 1984 won't be like *Nineteen Eighty-Four*"). The then-LA-based agency behind it had even put together video interviews with the creative team. So I just speak to the account exec over the phone, watch the video, and type my article on my new electronic typewriter—an early word processor with miniscule memory.

My article runs on the front page.

***

After four articles of decreasing length and prominence, however, the freelance assignments dry up. Dave says his budget is shot but recommends me to a trade-magazine publisher. For the next few years I'm writing puff pieces for magazines with titles like *Tradeshow Manager* and *Rx Home Care*. (Yes, that includes wheelchair dealerships.) I never let on about my disability. It's all done by phone, mail, and fax.

Until one day my cover is blown.

The editor says there's a staff opening. I apply. I've been working for her for at least a year, so I show up brimming with self confidence. She takes a hard look at me across her crowded desk and, after some chit-chat, asks, "How would you make photocopies?"

I smile to cover my surprise. Calmly, I explain how it's not hard to find someone to push a button for me, if necessary. I explain that I'm especially good at handling myself, that my disability has never held me back. I'm competent and can cope.

"But if we hire you," she says, "you'd be here to help *us*, not for us to help *you*."

Needless to say, I don't score the position. She likes my work enough to keep feeding me freelance assignments; she just doesn't want me around the office.

I've spent my life reassuring people that I'm okay, that I can do things that might surprise them. But all of a sudden this tactic is failing. It seems Mom was wrong. I can't really be anything I want now that I've grown up.

***

One night ML and I come home late to our dinky Rampart apartment. The ramp—around back, off a short dark alley—is covered in cockroaches. It's pitch black out. While she's fumbling for her keys I hear a scuffle and a thud. I can't see what's going on, but ML is on the ground. She hops up suddenly and is hollering.

"Give me back my purse! Come back here, you bastard!"

She tears off down the street. Her soprano voice is loud, projectile, and apartment windows above us open. I see a woman's head emerge from one of the windows. "Police," I say. "Call the police." But I'm not loud, or she doesn't speak English or want to get involved.

ML comes back and breathlessly explains she was knocked down and her purse snatched. I have a vivid imagination and a burning fear of her getting raped that's probably one part love and two parts physical insecurity. The movie in my head of another man being physically aggressive with her taunts me more and more.

But this night ML says she's fine; she's not hurt and wasn't "violated," just robbed. Later, the police will say that being knocked down does count as an assault. For the moment, though, the guy who took her purse took everything. She'd been holding my wallet as well as hers. From then on, I start carrying a small zippered pouch inside my chair.

The only thing she has left is the set of keys clutched in her hand. We decide it's unsafe to stay in our apartment. The robber has her driver's license with the address, and my set of keys. He could be back. So we call ML's brother in the Valley, and he sets us up at a local motel.

A week later—after less than a year in the Rampart District—we rent a larger, more expensive, safer apartment on LA's West Side.

***

At around this time, in St. Louis, Missouri, Virginia (Gini) Laurie—daughter of a surgeon and sister of a young man who died of polio, but not disabled herself—launches the International Polio Network (later called Post-Polio Health International). One of its key accomplishments will be spreading awareness of Post Polio Syndrome, in which people who'd contracted the condition decades earlier suddenly face new physical limitations—their joints and muscles, in effect, age more rapidly than other people's.

A similar effect will be found in SMA survivors, too—like me.

My self-esteem plummets as reality seems to close in around me. Anywhere ML and I go, at any time (even to this day), we can be side-winded by a stranger's inquisitiveness: *Is he your brother? Is she your nurse? Is he your son?* (Ouch!) Back on the multicolored streets of New York, I was one of many characters in public view; New Yorkers pride themselves on not being surprised by anything. But here, among the beautiful people, I feel awkward and ill fitting. Waiters overlook me and ask her what *he'll* be ordering. I remember one mostly empty restaurant where the manager came out to tell us there were no tables available, and practically chased us out the door!

For the most part these affronts roll off. But sometimes they sting. It's not true, of course, that my childhood in New York was without such comments. But where I used to be praised as heroic, inspirational, or angelically cute, I now feel insulted.

Some folks, out-of-the-blue, dub ML a saint—others, conversely, let on that I *must* be wealthy (or she would've fled by now). Fortunately, we've been enlightened by reading the *Disability Rag* and recognize what's going on. That it's not just us, or something wrong with us, but something wrong with *them*. So instead of driving a wedge between us, the occasional barrage of prejudicial horseshit brings us closer. It gives us a common enemy. Again, we two against the world!

In 1986, when I'm twenty-three, we're only beginning to understand we're part of something bigger. That year, the National Council on the Handicapped will publish a report called "Toward Independence," which will argue that federal legislation is sorely needed to protect the civil rights of disabled people. For people like me, this study will clarify two important points: (1) you probably have been discriminated against, your civil rights violated; (2) there's nothing you can do about it because, in most cases, discrimination against the disabled is still perfectly legal.

***

Through all these tensions, ML never bugs me about my under-employment. She sees how hard I'm working to find work. Plus we've wisely kept our finances separate. I don't depend on her financially at all. Just emotionally. In the midst of prejudice and isolation, I lean on her for the validation of love, of connection. And, yes, of sex.

As soon as she comes home from the chaotic classroom where she teaches, I pounce on her with requests, with demands for attention (like a two-year-old, only nowhere near as cute). With a few minor adjustments she can get me more comfortable in my chair than the attendant could all day. Plus I need to tell her every thought I've had since the morning—and pump her for information about her day, about the outside world. I don't have the interactions, the feedback, of the employed. In Los Angeles it's too easy to become isolated. It's easy for a writer to become isolated, too. And when you add in a disability, that's a perfect trifecta for the desolation of loneliness.

I'm twenty-three and still financially dependent on Dad. He pays for the attendant, my health insurance, and any medical expenses it doesn't cover. Other than that, I'm earning $5,000 a year, at best, from freelance writing, and still receive about three hundred a month from Social Security—now that the SSI debt is paid off—and several hundred more from property and stocks I've inherited. Because my combined savings exceeds a measly two thousand dollars, I'm deemed too rich to qualify for Medicaid.

I recall how Dean Crooks at Harvard had said my father must be rich as Croesus; I didn't understand at the time, but maybe Crooks was right. Though that's not the way Dad's behaving. He always seems worried about money—at once generous and tightfisted. Definitely a mixed message. Every three or four months he visits. To him it's a show of concern, of love. But I can't help feeling he's checking on his investment—in me. And time after time I'm just not measuring up.

Before every visit, I get the carpets cleaned, hire a maid service, take the van to be hand-detailed, and cut my hair. He never notices. At fifty-nine years old, he always wants to take us out to "somewhere nice." Because he once lived in LA, Dad thinks he knows the town. He takes us to Tail o' the Cock, Scandia, The Windsor, Musso & Frank Grill, the Polo Lounge . . . high-priced eateries of yesteryear. When I'm trying to learn to live on a budget. Yup, mixed message.

"I could take you under my wing," he says grandly, vaguely, at almost every turn, "but the financial world can be so dry—you don't want to do hackwork."

Dad's freelancing for financial magazines, fund managers, and firms. It's steady, well-paid work he constantly derides, belying his fantasies of doing something greater—and, it's clear to me now, revealing his state of disappointment and depression. At the time, though, I'm left wondering if I'm supposed to contradict or agree.

I start saying maybe. "How can I know, Dad, how I'll feel about financial journalism? I've never tried."

This doesn't move him, however. He was just talking theoretically . . . pie in the sky. But there's an element of blame in his voice. On some level he thinks I'm at fault for my chronic under-employment. He wants to help but is grasping at straws, desperately trying to be a good provider—a provider of ideas, not just money. My failure is his failure.

Actually, what he's doing is what I used to do—failing to recognize the extent of my disability, and employers' squeamishness about it.

(Alec, on the other hand, is earning a master's in applied social research and has "a good career ahead of him" in political and market surveying, proclaims Dad. Though Dad doesn't say it, the implication is clear, at least to me: Why are you, Ben, having such a hard time finding a job?)

One Sunday brunch, for no particular reason, Dad wants to take us to the Hotel Bel-Air. "If you've never been, it's something special," he explains.

ML's had enough of his fancy restaurants and claims a migraine. But I've never been there and I'm curious. Dad hasn't been there in decades, but he remembers it fondly. I think, too, he's looking for some place in LA where men have to wear a jacket and tie. He's quite obsessed with dress codes—perhaps a holdover from his *GQ* days?—and frequently laments LA's lack thereof.

As my weekend attendant, ML dresses me in my one suit, a button-down shirt, and a favorite conservative necktie. Then she relaxes with the Sunday paper while Dad drives the van along winding Sunset Boulevard to Stone Canyon. It's a lovely, clear fall day as we pull up to the hotel. Undeniably beautiful, the grand old place's lush grounds—the stream, the swans, the thick green foliage. It's like another land. You can forget you're in the middle of an urban desert.

Inside, we head for the small, darkened restaurant. Is there music—a piano? a harp?—or is that just an atmospheric tone my memory has created? It's practically empty, and the few men there are indeed in business attire even on a late Sunday morning. I remember ordering tortilla soup because it's something I'd never heard of; also, the word "tortilla" doesn't seem to go with the place's formality, a contrast that appeals.

Recently, as feeding myself has become more difficult than ever, I've discovered I do best if my elbows stick firmly in one place on the armrests of my wheelchair. To hold the right position, I need to push up my sleeves and bare my elbows; skin sticks to the upholstery better than fabric. Of course, doing this now will ruin my look—my suit-and-tie look, that is.

"Dad," I say, trying to be more attuned to and assertive of my needs and wishes, "I'd like to push up my sleeves. Do you suppose I can get away with that here?"

"Oh, I don't think so."

He's dead serious, which to me is the wrong answer. Granted I'd set him up—posed my request as a question. My therapist wouldn't have approved. But it was a rhetorical question. A joke, sort of. I'd wanted him to say, "Of *course* you can. Who cares what anybody else thinks!" He'd blown his line, his opportunity to step up to defend me and, by extension, the rights of all disabled people—proving he's more concerned with formality and appearances, with authority and making a good impression, than with my comfort, my need for a reasonable accommodation. To me, it's a betrayal, a disavowal of my community, my newfound disability consciousness.

"No, seriously, I need to," I say. I explain how it improves my ability to eat. And he complies. He pushes up my sleeves so I can feed myself.

I make a mental note to bring ML here sometime. It really is a lovely place.

The next day, or perhaps on a subsequent visit, he says, "Maybe I'm giving you too much money."

It's almost as if Dad, sitting cross-legged before me at the small glass-circle-topped table in our new one-bedroom apartment, is thinking aloud. The cheap table wobbles as if from the impact of his words. The implication is that financial support is somehow robbing me of motivation. Which is untrue. The logical corollary, then, is that I'd have a job if only I tried harder. Also untrue. What's worse, pressuring me—making me feel bad—doesn't inspire me to work better, to think more creatively.

After building me up at the Hotel Bel-Air, he now makes me want to shrivel up and disappear.

***

The discrepancy—the rift—between Dad's perceptions and my view of reality seems so stark and unbridgeable that I become downright stupefied and tongue-tied. Dad still holds such natural authority it makes me doubt myself, my instincts.

When he's gone, when I'm alone or with ML, my instincts tell me louder and louder that the culprit is disability prejudice. I'm heartened in 1987 by the best actress Oscar bestowed on Marlee Matlin (no relation) for *Children of A Lesser God*, which single-handedly makes sign language and the name "Mattlin"—no matter how many T's—look cool. And a year later, when students at Gallaudet University, the school for Deaf people, in Washington, DC, pull off a week-long campus shutdown to protest the installation of a new university president who is not hearing-impaired—and win!—I know it's important and right.

I know things are changing. More profoundly, I know that whether I like it or not I am part of that change. I've never been political, but a sense of discrimination is blazing around me like a burning bush, and I know I must respond. I must become involved.

In 1988, when I'm twenty-four, Congressman Tony Coelho and Senator Lowell Weicker introduce a bill outlawing discrimination against people like me in all aspects of society—not just at publicly funded schools and organizations. For the first time in my life, I write to Congress to urge passage.

The following year, the President's Committee on Employment of the Handicapped is renamed the President's Committee on Employment of People with Disabilities—followed a few months later by the renaming of the Education for All Handicapped Children Act as the Individuals with Disabilities Education Act. What's in a name? Not much. But even I learn to say "people with disabilities" instead of "the handicapped." It's an awkward phrase, but it *is* the one chosen by the vanguard of the movement so I respect it. Not because of the sanctimonious "people first" movement, or the bogus etymology that claims the word *handicap* comes from the idea of begging with hand in cap. (It doesn't.) Linguistically speaking, the oldest and arguably most accurate term is "cripple," which some disability-rights leaders take on as a kind of in-your-face badge of pride. In time, I do too.

One of those leaders becomes a fast friend. Her name is Barbara (just like my stepmother), and she's starting a local group for Jews with disabilities. To me, this sounds tailor-made for getting me out and meeting people (as I've said, LA is a notoriously difficult city for meeting people). In our first phone conversation, I'm struck by the pauses in her voice as she takes puffs from a ventilator. I'm also dead certain she doesn't want my sympathy. "*Ach*, life is tough for everybody," she tosses off.

What really floors me is when she says she has spinal muscular atrophy, too. I've never met anyone who shares my diagnosis.

She invites me to a gathering of friends with disabilities—Jews and gentiles. I've never really socialized with other disabled people, but I say yes.

When I meet her face to face, I'm surprised Barbara is so attractive. Wide, soulful eyes and thick, cascading red hair, not the angry hag I guess I'd imagined—not someone who's rejected society before it can reject her. In fact, she's an elegant, pencil-thin woman who's only recently taken to using a motorized wheelchair. The chair has a beeping portable ventilator attached. She has a lot more physical strength than I do, except when it comes to breathing. She drives her own van and can even walk a few steps. She lives on her own.

Spinal muscular atrophy, I learn, comes in many forms.

In time Barbara invites us to a series of dinners and meetings. I become a kind of project for her. At one of the first dinners—at Barbara's smart, new, government-subsidized accessible apartment—ML and I are introduced to another way of life. Several other ways, actually. Some people are fed by assistants, who stand over them quietly. Another feeds himself with his feet. A dapper man at the opposite end of the table asks to have the *position* of his food identified. "Chicken is at six o'clock, squash at four o'clock, and your wine is at ten o'clock." Whenever people address him, they identify themselves first. As in, "Hi. It's Ben." His guide dog (note: nobody says "seeing-eye dog") sits quietly at his feet.

The energetic conversation whipping around the crowded room is not whiny and small but upbeat, expansive, sarcastic, and overwhelmingly political. These people don't just bear their disabilities but bare them—flaunt them with pride.

ML and I, both social chameleons, take all this in poker-faced. We're acquiring a new etiquette. To be honest, though, I can't help but feel like I've stumbled upon a circus freak show. That's partly because it's *all* people with disabilities. Wall to wall crips!

ML is the only guest—as opposed to the few hired assistants—who doesn't limp or stagger or anything. She doesn't mind socializing with my new gang—at least to a point. She's not too fond of the droolers, though— hey, everyone has limits—and resents it when people assume she's a sort of designated AB ("able-bodied"), ever available to assist with personal tasks like emptying someone's leg bag. What would these people have done if she weren't there?

Yet for me there is a magnetic pull. Have I found my long-lost tribe? Is this the cure for my existential loneliness? Among them, can I stop pretending I'm a gainfully employed yuppie? Can I stop feeling bad about not being one? I recall my mother's repeated advice, and understand at last why she encouraged me to spend time with other disabled children.

An odd thing about this new milieu of mine: It's pretty clear who the enemy is. Nondisabled people, often referred to as TABs, for Temporarily Able-Bodied, may be useful when you need them. But when it comes to the struggle for autonomy and equality, they are definitely the oppressors.

＊＊＊

My new friends ask me to write an op-ed against the Jerry Lewis telethon. Barbara says I'm the best one to do it because I'm an ex-poster child.

There's an offensive piece in *Parade* magazine ostensibly written by Lewis as he tries to imagine himself in a wheelchair. It's the usual drivel, but Barbara says it must be answered. She introduces me to Paul Longmore, a historian of all things disability. I already know his name from articles I've read. He's famous for publicly burning his own book, in protest, when his earnings led Social Security to cut his benefits.

Paul gets me up to speed on the history of disability as a social construct—and I'll never see the world the same way again. First, he says, came the "moral model" of disability—physical deformity as a sign of spiritual decay and sin. Any number of villains come to mind. The Phantom of the Opera, Captain Hook, Long John Silver, etc. Then came the more enlightened "medical model"—disabled people are victims, not villains. They shouldn't be feared but pitied, helped, healed, cured. Best example: Tiny Tim.

In the 1970s came the revolutionary "civil-rights model," in which people with disabilities began to define themselves and advocate for their rights.

Thus inspired, I write an essay I call "An Open Letter to Jerry Lewis," pleading with him to change his offensive ways. I overnight my piece to the *New York Times*—the only paper that matters, according to my upbringing—and it's accepted. Unfortunately, news events—especially Iraq's invasion of Kuwait—intervene and my essay is canceled. A year later the LA *Times* publishes a revised version.

***

Barbara also introduces me to Kelly. Kelly is a dynamic woman who's only about four feet tall. I find her deep maple-syrup voice, pleading eyes, and soft hands seductive—and she encourages me to, pressing herself close, holding my hand at gatherings. Only later do I discover that's because she and the guy she's living with are having problems and she wants to make him jealous.

Could ML really ever understand me, not being disabled herself? I find myself wondering. Have I made a wrong turn somewhere? Did I go for ML as a kind of mother substitute all those years ago, and now need a more mature relationship?

My infatuation with Kelly is short-lived, but for a time I feel genuinely tempted to cheat on ML. I have something to prove—something about my attractiveness, my freedom and mobility. I need to know I'm with ML because I want to be, not because I have to be. Not because I'm stuck.

When we talk about it, ML says, "I hope she's good for you."

Later, after the evil temptation has passed, we skirt around the issue of our interdependence and the pressure it's brought to bear. She says we're both stuck, in a way. "But that's not necessarily a bad thing," she says. We owe a lot to necessity. If I left her, I'd be stuck until I made other attendant arrangements. At the same time, she can't leave me because she knows I depend on her. "But that keeps us together, gets us through the rough patches," she says.

"I don't want our relationship to be based on obligation," I protest.

I know it to be true, though—our interdependence has become oppressive. This is partly why I've thrown myself into the disability-rights movement, why I'm so attracted to people with whom I have no dependency issues.

We're talking in our apartment. I've turned around from the table where I've set up a computer, speakerphone, and tape recorder. I've worked out a system for the computer. It involves using the eraser end of an unsharpened pencil, for leverage. Sometimes I copy and paste individual letters from one document to another, to make entering text easier. It's a slow process but I derive a tremendous sense of accomplishment and autonomy from it.

ML is leaning on the kitchen counter. It's a tiny kitchen, but then there's just the two of us. Which is part of the problem. I'm still completely reliant upon her at night and on weekends. It's become a bad habit—one I suspect we're both afraid to break.

I wonder aloud if I ought to hire more assistants.

"But then we'd have to deal with *them*," she groans in such a way that we both chuckle.

She's never liked any of my attendants. She says she can do the job better, which is true. Nobody has ever cared for me better than she does. But her resentment of them is self-defeating. Can't she see that her solicitousness reinforces my dependence on her . . . and generally undermines my sense of autonomy? I may not like the attendants either, but they're essential to my maintaining a separate life and so, sometimes, I *make* myself find something to like about them.

Then again, I must acknowledge I don't know anymore why things are the way they are. Do I lean on her too much, my spine turned to mush? Or has she become addicted to my needing her?

"Besides," she continues, "even when I'm *not* here—when I'm at work—I still feel responsible. None of them is really all that capable or reliable." She pauses, reaches toward me, and abruptly pulls out one of my eyebrow hairs. "Was about to fall into your eye," she explains as if it were the most ordinary gesture in the world.

It may be true, but she has to stop doing that, stop invading my personal space, stop mothering me. And I have to stop letting her. That is, if I can make her stop.

At the moment, the attendant is particularly bad—which tends to feed the problem, to make me cling to her all the more (and make her exhausted compensating for his shortcomings). When Peter didn't show up one morning—and his roommate said he'd packed up and disappeared, owing a month's rent—I'd hired a new guy from an agency: Sunday. That's his name. (Truthfully.) He says his father is a Nigerian tribal chieftain (why do these guys always need to impress me with how important they used to be?) who had no less than twenty-five wives and eighty-five children . . . and they just ran out of names.

I think because of Kenny—my old high school helper and pal—I'm prejudiced in favor of Black guys. I liked Sunday at the beginning. He's tidy and clean, wears nonprescription glasses for cosmetic purposes, and is full of outsize ambitions. But the relationship has deteriorated. He's showing up late in the morning, making foolish excuses, and failing at routine errands (again with absurd explanations).

There was one early sign of weirdness, come to think of it. Doing our laundry, he announced he wouldn't wash ML's bras and panties—couldn't even remove them from the hamper! "It is a custom among my people. I am forbidden to touch women's undergarments," he explained.

By this point, I'm looking for an excuse to fire him. Still, I need to know I *can* cope without ML. That I could find a better attendant—a team of them—and survive on my own, if necessary. Not have to go back and move in with Dad, which has become one of my biggest fears.

But then, am I with her—do I occasionally appease her—simply because she's the best helper I've ever had or ever will have? Back when I agreed to let her do helpful tasks for me, was it our romance's death knell? Is it too late to rectify our love?

"You're not so perfect yourself," I say, for lack of a better comeback, still blinking from her impromptu plucking.

We have a joke that we would've broken up long ago but our fights are so damn clever and enjoyable. This time, mine is a poor showing.

"Look, I don't want to leave. Where would I go?" she says. "Besides, if the fact that you need me keeps us from breaking up—if it sort of forces us to work out our differences—maybe that's a good thing."

We agree that if we're still together in three years we'll get married. We shop for a cheap diamond ring and everything. I just don't want to tie the knot before I'm twenty-five, and I imagine she doesn't want to turn thirty still single. This cockeyed logic somehow makes sense to both of us.

***

In August 1989—when I'm twenty-six and she's twenty-nine—we have a small, interfaith wedding at a hotel in West Hollywood. (The Bel-Air was too expensive.) I'll never forget how . . . when I first see her in all her bridal finery . . . even after six years' living together . . . her magnetic chocolate-brown eyes, firm cheekbones, and soft pouty-smiling lips snatch my breath away. (One of those clichés that's spot-on accurate.)

Our families gather around, toast us with champagne, and make a few speeches. In his toast, Alec says, "I'm glad Ben's found someone to take care of him."

Ugh!

(At least I think that's what he says. His actual words may have been "someone to care for him.")

Shortly after, we travel East to share our wedding album with family who couldn't make it. In Baltimore, I'm particularly pleased to see Great Aunt Sarah—a thin, tirelessly warm-hearted favorite of mine who must be well into her nineties at this point.

"Look at you," she says slowly, seated in a high-backed chair beside me, reaching a spidery hand toward my inanimate one. "Look at you. Paula's miracle baby!"

"Oh, come on—"

"You *are*. To think how she cried when you were small . . . You weren't supposed to live. You *are* a miracle. Paula's miracle baby."

Contemplating this after, I shrink away from the absurdity of it. The responsibility—being a miracle is a burden, a burden I don't need. And yet, *am* I a miracle baby . . . all grown up?

A year after our wedding, the Americans with Disabilities Act is signed into law. It doesn't end "disability oppression." It doesn't get me a job. But it tells ML and me that we're not alone in the stresses we've been facing. They're real, I haven't imagined them, and they're not fair.

CHAPTER NINE

BECOMING MORE DISABLED

1992-1995

> "Life is a tragedy filled with suffering and despair and yet some people do manage to avoid jury duty."
> —Woody Allen, in the *New York Times*,
> October 16, 2011

It's Super Bowl Sunday—a fact I'm only dimly aware of, not being a football fan—and we're sleeping late. We've moved to a two-bedroom condo down the block; the second bedroom is my office, at least until there are children to fill it. The down payment for which came mostly from liquidating the stocks I'd purchased after selling the New York apartment, and partly from Dad— what he'd elusively and morbidly called "an advance on inheritance." We had the doorways widened for better wheelchair access—perhaps the chief benefit of home ownership.

When we're both sufficiently awake to communicate on this chill February morning, I ask ML to roll me onto my back. Nothing unusual in that. It's my wake-up position—suitable for watching TV, drinking coffee, making love, or just cuddling, etc.

This particular morning, it seems it'll be coffee and TV. Except something feels wrong. My right leg is . . . asleep, maybe? Semi-numb. All tingly. Probably slept on it funny. It'll go away, I figure, and don't mention it until later— when I tire of the Sunday morning TV preachers (though their methods of communication I find fascinating) and infomercials for luxury real estate.

"Can you move my right leg, please?" I say. "Turn it over, to the outside . . ."
She does what I ask. The icy exoskeleton sensation remains unmoved.

Still, I do not panic. Waking up with a numb limb isn't entirely new to me. There have been mornings I arise with a hand that feels comically swollen, like Wile E. Coyote's paw after it's been smashed under a ten-ton boulder. The result of sleeping with my head on my hand. Always fades in a few hours.

And as a kid, I recall, I had many such strange spells—the inexplicable "fireballs" that intermittently and invisibly pummeled my skin one summer, cured only by mysterious capsules prescribed by a Fire Island doctor—a placebo, I suspect now—followed months later by a flu-related sensory episode I called "the flat feeling" that temporarily twisted my perceptions of textures and surfaces. Both never explained—chalked up to a combination of childhood imagination and my wacky neurological makeup.

This time it's my entire leg, from the groin down . . . the extent of which I slowly realize as ML washes me. But she's so used to my kvetching about minor discomforts—my position in the wheelchair, say, or sinus irritation due to changing weather—that she scarcely pays attention to my tentative complaint.

Once I'm up, on the phone with Barbara—my ambassador to the disability community, not my stepmother—I ask if she's ever experienced a tingling numbness like this. (Speakerphone-to-speakerphone conversations are tricky, since they only communicate one way at a time. Whichever end is louder drowns out the other. Fortunately, we're both used to this phenomenon and diligently take turns.)

"Freaky," she says. "Life with *smah*. . . ." (She's referring to spinal muscular atrophy, or SMA.)

"But it's not supposed to affect sensory nerves, just motor nerves," I say.

"Doctors can be a great resource, but don't believe them all the time."

I've been brought up to trust doctors like they're Holy People, but I have to admit I'm finding the insights of other folks with disabilities like mine much more valuable. And given the dubious tradition of nondisabled people speaking for the disabled—clinicians, writers, politicians—it's eye-opening to talk with someone who's been there, who shares your perspective.

That afternoon ML and I go to her brother's new house in Chatsworth. It's a big Victorian-style number, and her whole family has gathered there. They spread out and sort of float between rooms; there is no organized, formal center, not with my in-laws. Conversation is similarly scattered and random, but unfailingly pleasant.

Eventually my father-in-law turns on the football game, and I sit and watch with him without much interest. Part of my problem is, I never learned the rules of football. As a kid I could hold a Wiffle-ball bat and get pushed around the bases, so I learned the basics of baseball. But football? Never.

And there, in front of the TV, in the deep-red-paisley-papered den, my right leg is throbbing worse than ever . . . and my left one is starting to get pins-and-needles, too.

I keep it to myself, but the sensation—thrumming and dull, not painful—is spreading.

***

"It's a neuropathy," says my physician. I'd called him first thing Monday morning, and he was able to see me that afternoon. To me, there are two kinds of doctors—those who merely go through the motions, who minimize your complaints and worries, never taking you seriously, and those who overreact, who treat you like you're in intensive care. I prefer the latter. These are doctors who make me feel like a VIP.

This particular doctor is an asthma expert, that being my chief ailment, but he's also an internist and the only doctor I've seen on a regular basis since moving to California nearly seven years ago. I trust him and like his occasionally gruff manner. He never shies away from giving a precise diagnosis, even if it's a bullshit term like *neuropathy*. (He's Dad's age and in fact was referred by Dad's internist in New York.)

"I'm going to give you a shot of vitamin B12," he says, "and if you don't feel better by tomorrow I'll refer you to a neurologist. Do you have a neurologist?"

"No," I say, thinking *not since Dr. Spiro back to New York*.

If you've never had it, I recommend B12 as a great pick-me-up. I leave his office feeling euphoric, with energy coursing through my veins. My new attendant, Jorge, whom I hired from the California unemployment office—a great new source of candidates, I hope—after Sunday left for Nigeria (and subsequently leveled a workman's comp claim for alleged back strain, which he'd only noticed a month after being replaced), drives me home. Jorge asks no questions. That's partly because he's too busy wolf whistling at women out the van window. (Another stereotype, I know, that's nonetheless true in this case.)

The tingling, now spread upward to my chest, continues undeterred.

That night, ML and I make love. (B12 is also a terrific aphrodisiac!) For me it's a weird experience. Afterward I timidly ask, "What just happened?"

"You don't know?"

"I think I came. Right? I'm pretty sure. But I'm not certain I'm feeling accurately."

This time ML does pay attention. She starts patting me down. "Can you feel this? And this?"

I *can* feel them—all her pats and pokes—but as if through a gauzy shield.

The next day the tingling has moved into my arms. I can no longer hold a pen or work the TV remote. I phone my doctor, who says I've probably pinched a nerve in my neck. My neck *is* weak and my head does flop about freely, given a push or jolt. And it's true that Jorge—a soft-hearted jock from Peru—is rough with me sometimes. Every morning he lifts me from bed to my wheelchair with a forceful herky-jerkiness and a grunt, as if I weighed two tons instead of just over a hundred-twenty pounds. It's a roughness I've encouraged. I've urged my attendants not to be too gentle, not to think of me as a delicate flower. "You're not going to hurt me," I'd reassure the first time they handle me, to keep them from babying me and ensure they move me about as needed. There is a degree of necessary roughness. But perhaps Jorge had taken my macho promptings too much to heart.

At the end of our morning routine I often feel winded and shaken, needing to collect myself at my desk before getting down to work. Yet I never say "ouch" or "stop—that's too rough," locked into some sort of masculine game of virility where I'm afraid to come out the wimp. I'd always told myself that the aftereffect, the necessity of realigning my wits, was like recovering from a jostling morning commute, nothing more. I wonder now if it's actually a sort of attendant-cripple version of Stockholm syndrome.

At my doctor's referral, I meet the next morning with a new neurologist—a nebbishy academic type with a harried, impatient manner. "Can you feel this?" he asks, holding a tuning fork to my right knee.

"Yes."

"Tell me when the vibrations stop."

I do, and he gives little indication of how well or poorly I've done but I suspect the gizmo is still vibrating after I can no longer feel it. He runs a few more tests and continues to seem dismissive. Or baffled. (I guess he'd go in

Category One of doctors I've known: one of the under-whelmed.) "There are a number of viruses that can cause this sort of neuropathology. Let's check for actual damage," he says and orders an MRI.

I expect his reaction might've been bigger if I actually used my legs. I mean, there's no big loss here. In truth, it's the loss of use of my hands that scares me.

So the next weekend—the first appointment I can get—I'm slid bodily into the giant MRI tunnel. As instructed, I lie still (not that I have much choice) to the sounds of banging microwaves or whatever they are. It occurs to me that the metal rods in my spine—the ones put in during that high school surgery—might skew this device's readings . . . since it's *Magnetic* Resonance Imaging. (I've written about modern imaging technologies for one of my med-equipment trade magazines.)

I also think of a joke while in there, which I hold onto until the ordeal is over. "Sounds like the bombing of Beirut in there," I say, back in my chair. I also mention my metal rods.

The technician doesn't laugh, and maybe makes a note about the rods. Mostly he's trying to diagnose me. "I'll bet it's Guillain-Barré!" he announces with a flourish of his arms, stumbling a moment over the French words. "What's your doctor say? Ask him if it's Guillain-Barré syndrome."

It's as if he thinks he'll win a gold star for finding someone with this diagnosis.

Isn't it what Joseph Heller recently recovered from? is what I'm thinking.

I never do get an official diagnosis. By the time I manage to get a hold of the neurologist, the tingling has already begun receding from my legs. Limb by limb the sensation fades. After two months, it vanishes completely, in the same manner in which it appeared.

Still, the neurologist sticks with the virus explanation—though he doesn't specify Guillain-Barré. Ultimately, it doesn't matter. It's gone.

But it's left behind a great deal of damage. I never regain the ability to hold a pencil or work the TV remote.

***

Two hours. Two and a quarter. First in a bland waiting room full of families with small, thin-limbed children, then in a claustrophobic examination room.

I'm here to see Dr. Engel. Or should I say the Great and Powerful Dr. Engel? Whose name I got from Barbara, my disability connection. She says he's famous in the SMA world, a leading spinal muscular atrophy expert. I'm here to find out why I'm weaker.

Before Dr. Engel will see me, though, I'm pre-examined by his associate, whose name I forget now. Nearly two and a half hours to see his lieutenant! On the other hand, the starter doctor is kind of cool—a tall, elegant man with a copper-colored complexion. Towering over me, he is kind and unrushed.

I tell him I'm concerned because for the first time in memory I'm losing strength. He nods, unimpressed. For me, this is a big deal to admit, to lower the Brave Face, stop pretending everything is normal—and yet I feel nothing but relief at his calm reaction. I didn't come here for sympathy, after all. I came for knowledge.

"When was your last EMG?" he asks.

I stutter a moment, then mutter something about having an EKG with my annual physical—

"No," he corrects, a smile softening his granite physiognomy. "I'm referring to an electro*myo*gram. Never, I'm guessing?"

Never even heard of it. Perceptive, he is.

After asking a few more questions, he leads me to another examination room and gently administers the EMG. I say "gently" because it's a savage procedure, involving small needles stuck up and down my arm—and zapping them one by one with a bolt of electricity. This somehow tests nerve reactions. I can remain in my chair and keep my clothes on, at least—so I've let Jorge stay in the waiting room. He gets claustrophobic and uncomfortable around doctors anyway.

Mine announces evidence of progression. Progression of the atrophy, that is. In other words, the opposite of progression. Worsening. "You have some degeneration here," he observes after a particularly strong set of shocks.

I ask how that's possible, protest that I thought my condition had stabilized when I was about six. "Are we even sure I *have* spinal muscular atrophy?" I ask as an arctic cloud wafts over and settles on my body.

"The atrophy can start up again with age, particularly with prolonged inactivity," the doctor explains, his tone steady, neutral. "It can stop and start anytime, honestly."

"I didn't know that. Is this a new discovery?"

"Not really."

So this is what it feels like to receive information that makes you reevaluate your entire life. Hit the rewind button and watch it all over again, looking for signs, for clues.

"Do you think it'll continue, this new round of weakening?" I soldier on, after a hard swallow. "How far will it go?"

"Can't say. But no, not necessarily. It can stop and start intermittently. In any case, it's gradual. Almost always the progression occurs gradually."

After a moment of taking this in, I'm reminded of those families in the waiting room—the scared ones with kids who are just being diagnosed, kids who might not live to their tenth birthdays. The chill cloud is theirs, not mine.

Anyway, didn't I already know I was growing weaker? Not really news, then, is it? "What about the tingling?" I ask. I describe my recent numbness, how it came suddenly, lingered for two months, and then disappeared just as suddenly.

"That's not spinal muscular atrophy, of course. Spinal muscular atrophy doesn't affect sensory nerves—"

"Yes. I know."

"—And your sensory nerves seem fine, by the way. So I don't know what the tingling you describe came from. But any prolonged inactivity could cause progression. Or it could be unrelated."

Doctors! They really don't know shit, do they?

Yet I try to keep him talking, don't want to forget anything, to get home and kick myself for neglecting to cover something crucial. Besides, it's better than the quiet of an empty examination room. "So . . . no predictions?"

"We're finding that people with SMA who live long enough often experience some progression as their muscles wear out," he goes on. "Like Post Polio Syndrome. Often people in their fifties go on ventilators for the first time in their lives, as breathing becomes too difficult."

"Great," I say. "Something to look forward to." It's all too much, and yet somehow not enough.

Later, I will research ventilator users, like Barbara. I will learn that even people who put it off as long as possible find using a vent is actually a great relief. They find they have more energy than before and only wish they'd made the switch earlier. A completely different perspective—one you can only get from talking to actual users.

Barbara will also say that SMA is an umbrella term used to describe a variety of scenarios. She herself used to walk, has only been using a chair and ventilator for the past few years. I'll ask her what it's like to lose functionality—how does one cope? Predictably practical and dismissive, she'll answer, "*Ach*, you have to plan ahead for it. And you mourn each loss, and then go on."

When Dr. Engel finally arrives, in my head I hear a fanfare like I've been granted an audience with royalty. (That's a joke—his full name is W. *King* Engel.) He's an average-size man with white hair, thick round glasses, and a bow tie—outwardly about as impressive as Orville Redenbacher—but he's bursting with energy and authority, or at least that's what I ascribe to him after the long buildup.

We review my medical history. He's very interested in my biography and what I'm doing now. I have a sense that much of the study of this condition is anecdotal, a collection of life stories in search of common traits or clues to the disease's origins and different strains.

"We're finding more and more cases of it around the world," he volunteers. "Egypt and Africa, Russia and Asia—you name it. It's not a rare condition." He's informing me like a professor more than a clinician. I'm oddly comforted by his air of intelligence—though his delivery isn't quite sugarcoated enough to qualify as good bedside manner, to my mind. He seems to respect my brains, too. We connect on an intellectual plane.

"But look at you," he says. "You're doing marvelously! Send me some of your writing, will you? I know someone who might be interested in meeting you."

I'm doing marvelously? I'm losing what little strength I've had! Compared to other cases he sees, however, I guess I'm still one of the lucky ones. I want to feel lucky again.

***

When I get home, I put together a package of writing samples and promptly send them to him. I include the LA *Times* op-ed that's critical of the Jerry Lewis telethon. I know Dr. Engel probably receives funding from the telethon, but I'm inclined to be completely candid with him.

A few weeks later he calls. My telethon essay reminds him of one of his other patients, he says—the one he'd mentioned wanting to introduce me to. Who turns out to be Evan Kemp, the Washington bigwig who'd written that groundbreaking anti-telethon op-ed in the *New York Times* more than a decade before. Kemp is now chairman of the US Equal Employment Opportunity Commission. He flies to LA periodically just to see Dr. Engel.

And this becomes the primary payoff of my visit to Dr. Engel. For in 1993, a little more than a year later, when Bill Clinton becomes president, Kemp will be out of a job. So he'll invest his personal fortune in launching a communications company about and for people with disabilities. Among other enterprises, his company will publish a monthly newspaper called *One Step Ahead*, and I'll be named its senior editor. I'll be put on retainer for half my time—spent mostly writing. My first regular paycheck. My first official employment contract and job title. But that's still a few years in the future.

First, I have to realign my life around my weakened (or possibly *weakening*) hands. Plan ahead, mourn the losses, and move on—that's what Barbara had said. Not that my hands ever did so much, but now I need extra help with everyday tasks. Such as eating. I've always had to be positioned just so to feed myself, but the "just so" position has become impossibly particular and fragile.

"Right elbow forward just a smidge . . . oh, too much . . . back a little . . ."

Some days I can't get it right at all.

It's not as if debility happens all at once. More and more it becomes simpler for ML to feed me dinner. It saves time, effort. Especially if I want to expand my diet beyond chicken nuggets—that is, beyond food that's easy to hold and stick in my mouth. If I want to try sushi, say, or sip soup, a greater degree of assistance is required.

At lunch, with Jorge, I still try to fake it as much as possible (that macho business). But I alter what I'm eating to make the assisted self-feeding go more smoothly. A slice of toast with a piece of cheese melted on it is fairly effortless to balance and shove in (whereas soft, untoasted bread collapses on itself). A cup of yogurt is easier to suck through a straw than eat by spoon, provided you've poured a dash of milk in. (I'd been drinking through straws since college, though I don't remember exactly when or why I give up lifting and tipping cups.)

Signs of my new weakness creep in elsewhere, too, like vermin. I begin allowing Jorge to brush my hair—telling him how I want it, rather than having him hand me the brush and support my arm aloft. Is it obvious, my "new look"?

He's not a stylist, and it's hard to explain brushstrokes—"back and right at a diagonal, toward my right ear . . ."

In high school I could spend hours primping at the mirror unassisted. Yes, often completely unassisted back then. Perhaps I'd been losing strength all along . . . incrementally, imperceptibly. If I ever thought about this, I told myself my arms had merely grown heavier over the years—that's why I sometimes needed more help than I used to. Plus I'm less interested in primping now, don't need to work at it.

Once weekend I receive a small package from Dad. He's transferred our old home movies from Super Eight to VHS cassette. He's titled it, "Alec & Ben: The Early Years."

Watching the silent images, I'm struck by the changes in my young body. As a baby I could crawl a little, even hold up my head. As a toddler I'm already concentration-camp thin, my movements awkward, tentative. Alec, by contrast, hogs the picture; he's always dancing, clapping his hands, showing his ability to be active, performing for the camera. Later still, when I'm maybe nine years old, I'm fatter and almost completely immobile from the neck down. I don't realize it at the time, I can see. But someone is always holding me, moving my arms. At a birthday party—a game of hot potato—I'm positioned in a circle with friends in our old living room, and the girl on my left puts the potato into my lap, where my hands are waiting, and then the boy on my right picks it up from there. I might think I'm passing it along, but in fact I'm completely passive.

Talking about this afterward, ML doesn't let me kid myself. I'd been almost thinking my new weakness was no biggie because I'd always been more debilitated than I knew or admitted. She says, almost apologetically, "I do miss your touch, your gentle caresses."

She's not characteristically one to express sorrow, disappointment, or need. She's a coper. She muddles through. She'd sooner ask what I want to do—and derive pleasure from doing that—than express a desire of her own. So I'm pleased she's being frank, but still her words sting.

"We just have to adapt," I say after a beat, unable to resist the find-a-solution orientation of my gender, or my upbringing. It's a glib response, the kind I'm preprogrammed for as part of my lifelong survival strategy. I do realize I'm hurt and scared, but do I realize it loud and clear enough to say so?

Yet even as the upwardly mobile, Harvard-educated man is evaporating—replaced by the severely disabled cripple—somehow I can't give up. You mourn and move on. It's a different direction but not a dead end. I'll have to adapt.

And on some dim level there's a glimmer that signals maybe I'll be better off. Maybe trying to fit in with the Harvard-yuppie ideal was unworkable and unrealistic.

Cripples are nothing if not full of creative solutions. I search for mine, for the best solutions to my current conundrums—not medical cures, mind you, on which I've long since given up. And which, at best, seem a long shot and, moreover, completely out of my control. Instead, I investigate everything from sex toys to revitalize our marital intimacy (did you know there's a whole catalog of sexual gear designed for the disabled?) to mechanical wheelchair attachments that might allow me greater arm movement.

I also search for intellectual comfort, for a solution to what psychologists might call my cognitive dissonance. And I find it, when I realize my increased limitations are, in part, a function of aging. Everybody ages. Everybody goes through diminished capacity as they grow older. So I make up a narrative I can live with: I may not be all I was when ML met me, say, but who is? To put it bluntly, she's aged, too. (Only later will I come to understand how much that very fact is simultaneously preying on ML's mind.)

***

In my search for the latest "adaptive" gear, as it's called, I attend the Abilities Expo. It's an annual tradeshow for the disability market—vans, high-tech wheelchairs that can stand you upright or climb stairs, telephone devices for the hearing impaired, fashionable attire for the seated or amputees, publications, benefits advocacy, and even a self-defense workshop for those with limited movement.

ML and I don't buy anything, but we collect a lot of flyers and ads. If we ever build our dream house, we now know where to acquire a bathtub with a watertight door for easy access, and kitchen cabinets that move up and down with the push of a button.

The Abilities Expo is just one of the places that make me feel good about my disability—where my so-called physical liabilities become assets. I become a volunteer board member at my local independent-living center, too, where I help with publications, do some fundraising, and participate in (and sometimes lead) discussion groups.

At one group presentation, in the Center's beige-on-beige community room, Paul Longmore—the disability historian—is explaining his disability-rights perspective on the right-to-die. He's against it, I know, but I'm curious because I thought disability rights was all about choice and self-determination.

"Question," I bark, after his presentation, because I can't raise my hand (I'm not the only one in the room who can't, either). "What if I'm really depressed? Say, my wife has left me, my brother's died in a horrible car accident, I've lost all my money and I have no job. I want to end it all but physically can't pull the trigger or give myself pills. Shouldn't I have the right to ask my attendant to help me commit suicide, without getting him in trouble?"

A silence echoes throughout the space. I feel like I've won a game of Stump the Expert. Then my friend Barbara, who's sitting beside Paul, trumpets, "That's different. I'll explain to you later, Ben."

It isn't the first time I've sensed the disability agenda to be somewhat rigid.

Once the crowd's dispersed, Barbara brings her chair close to mine. She says that, to the outside world, suicide could seem a rational choice for someone like her or me. After all, our shared diagnosis *is* terminal in many cases. "Anybody else contemplating suicide would receive intervention, because they're assumed to be depressed and treatable. But you and me ...? Society is too quick to allow cripples to off themselves," she says.

In fact, society sometimes seems to encourage disabled people to get out of the way, stop being a burden or stop using up scarce resources, she goes on. It can push disabled people to the margins, where they naturally become depressed. And instead of identifying their depression as treatable—instead of creating opportunities that make their lives worth living—society (she calls it "the majority culture") wants to push for the right to die before it's established the right to live.

"You know about Jack Kevorkian, right?" she asks. "How he takes advantage of newly diagnosed people to feed his own sick death wish."

It's a perspective I'd never garnered before, and I take it to heart. A few years later I'll try explaining it to the local chapter of the Hemlock Society, after the chapter head hears me give testimony at a state hearing on a proposed assisted-suicide bill, and invites me to address his clan. It's probably in vain, but I'll be paid fifty dollars for my troubles. One stalwart—a wiry, buzz-cut man in a gray cardigan, who opts to orate from a standing position—will reinforce my point by admitting the group advocates legalizing suicide for the terminally ill only as "a first step, because it's more palatable to the American public." What this crowd is really after, he concedes, is "a dignified death for everybody who wants it."

"*That* I could support," I say. "At least it's not discriminatory." I've become so comfortable with this subject—by then I've published another, related op-ed in the LA *Times* and am a card-carrying, T-shirt-owning member of Not Dead Yet—that I find myself waxing philosophic. "Don't you see that if the life of someone with a severe diagnosis is held more cheaply than someone else's, it has the effect of diminishing *all* people with disabilities? And if we're devalued any further, more of us *will* give up!"

Around the same time, I'm asked to join a workshop at LA's Mark Taper Forum to develop new theater pieces that advance the budding notions of Disability Culture and Disability Pride. For a month of Saturdays I brainstorm with other writers with disabilities—poets, essayists, playwrights, most in wheelchairs. We discuss Randolph Bourne, the early-twentieth-century intellectual who struggled against prejudice because of his twisted spine. We discuss a Depression-era protest group called the League of the Physically Handicapped, who objected to unfair treatment from the WPA. And, of course, we consider FDR himself, and his need to manipulate public perceptions of his disability.

I contribute a monologue about my experiences as an MDA poster child—which I'm later gratified to see performed on stage along with other consciousness-raising skits.

I also get up to speed on disability portrayals in movies and on TV. I'm asked to help pick the year's best for the Media Access Awards. I spend a Saturday afternoon in a hotel conference room in Universal City viewing clips—where I form a warm friendship with Robert David Hall, the disabled actor soon to enjoy success as a regular on *CSI*.

But separately—unconnected with the Media Access Awards—I part with the monolith of disability-rights opinion over the movie *My Left Foot*. A fine bit of filmmaking, to be sure, but I'm uncomfortable with its heavy-handed portrayal of disability and embarrass myself in a meeting at the independent-living center to discuss it. Someone declares the flick a marvel, the first true-to-life story from a disability perspective, which has become the sort of official party line. "Well, not *all* disabled people agree about that," I say for no particular reason except to assert my individuality.

A minor point of disagreement, perhaps, it will mark the beginning of my disillusionment with the movement.

***

Separately, my friend Barbara recommends a counselor in California's vocational-rehabilitation office. Heeding her advice—she speaks in her small voice with such authority!—I meet the advisor in his tiny office . . . a slight, intense man with unruly bushels of black-gray hair . . . and explain that I want Dragon Dictate.

I had seen this awe-inspiring device demonstrated a few years earlier in a laboratory at the California State University in Northridge. But you had to speak excruciatingly slowly into a special microphone—pausing. After. Every. Word. It would translate the sound into computer text, but was still utterly impractical. The thing filled a small room and cost about ten thousand dollars (the computer that worked with it went for another ten thousand).

By the time I'm requesting the state's financial aid to buy one, it's come down to four-thousand and can be installed on most regular PCs. "I'll buy the computer," I propose, "if the state can buy the software. It's necessary for my work."

In those days, California still has funds for this kind of investment. So within a few months a technician comes to my apartment to install Dragon Dictate and offer quick training. Today, of course, you can buy the latest version for about a hundred bucks—with built-in training. And it's geometrically faster and more accurate. Back then, though, for me at least, at nearly thirty, the advent of voice-recognition computing is nothing short of miraculous. Finally, an answer to how I'd interact with a keyboard with sufficient rapidity (as at least one would-be employer had inquired)!

It proves the right tool for the job, though not the paid kind. In two months I write a three-hundred-page novel. It's my second, actually; the first one—an embarrassing Bildungsroman about how a disabled young man's physical dependency complicates his struggle for autonomous adulthood, titled *Learning To Crawl*, after the Pretenders album—took five years and a hired typist to complete. The new one, a Hemingway-esque melodrama about a yuppie couple considering parenthood, called *The Baby Chase*, contains no mention of disability—in a cynical, failed attempt to boost its chances of publication. (Both manuscripts remain in dusty boxes on my shelf.)

Dragon opens a world to me that'll include the Internet, of course—a completely accessible means of not just socializing but doing research, which

I always found problematic in traditional libraries. In short, I'm no longer excluded from the computer revolution.

***

"Here kitty, kitty, kitty," ML calls out from the terrace to the feral cats in the neighboring apartment's courtyard. Her voice takes on a baby-talk quality when she comes inside and says, "I want something small to take care of."

This, or something like it, happens morning after morning.

Then, when we're out walking in the neighborhood, she accosts a bouncing toddler who's joyfully making his escape from his tired-looking nanny: "Excuse me, young man, but your shoes are untied."

The final tea-leaf revelation comes when she tells me her OB/GYN recommends a particular brand of ovulation predictor.

I know she went off the pill when we moved to the condo. She'd said she wasn't ready for kids yet but had heard "it can take five years to get all the pill out of you." Somehow, baby fever has come more quickly than expected—ask not for whom the biological clock tolls.

"I'm thirty-two," she reminds me, when showing the OvuQuick she'd purchased. "I'm already past my prime. Motherhood is slipping away!"

And so we begin the process. I'm fully functional sexually. No obvious explanation why she's not pregnant, after several months of basal-temperature taking and OvuQuick. The stresses quickly compound. ML can't shake the sense of inadequacy, of defeat. That her mother first became pregnant in her mid-twenties, and her younger sister already has three kids, adds a bitter flavoring to her emotional salmagundi.

Call it a crip thing, but I start out sure we'll find a solution if we're patient enough. Your body betraying you? Find a technology, a treatment, a creative workaround, a funding source—whatever it takes to accomplish your goals.

We venture together to a pantheon of fertility doctors. We learn I have a low sperm count—that's the diagnosis. Doubtless it's due to my sitting all day—or, it occurs to me, my frequent X-rays as a child. I recall many an X-ray technician when I was growing up who dismissed the notion of my ever fathering children and, therefore, needing a lead shield over my privates. Unless one of my parents was there to insist, it didn't happen.

Used to seeking medical expertise, to forcing my body to do things it doesn't naturally do, I feel no hesitation about beginning hormone treatments.

First pills. Then injections. Gonadotropin (trivia: it's made from the urine of postmenopausal nuns!) is so expensive (and not covered by insurance) that we drive to Tijuana to snag the vials cheap. We find a favorite motel in La Jolla to spend the night, and try to make the best of a bad thing. We have to make the trip multiple times.

On one such adventure we're stopped by a border guard. "Do you have a doctor's prescription for this?"

"No. Not on us. But he did send us here for it." Which is true.

The uniformed immigration Gestapo stares us down and repeats his single message: "You have to have a doctor's prescription."

In memory, I pride myself on breaking the standoff. I say to the guard as flatly and self-confidently as I can muster, "So what do we do?"

And I'll be damned if he doesn't back down! "Oh, I'll let you through. This time."

In fairness, ML's version of this—and of the four and a half grueling years we spend in the dark maze of infertility, the seemingly endless cycle of monthly disappointment followed by the fragile, tentative rebirths of hope—would surely be different from mine. But to me, she becomes hopelessly sullen and withdrawn, as if she's stumbled down a bottomless well.

About three years into the ordeal, to maximize our odds, ML starts hormone treatment to increase her egg production. (She has to give herself the injections.) One Saturday morning during this time, we go to the hospital for the egg retrieval. I pace the halls in my motorized wheelchair for the several hours she's in surgery—only I can't take it. It's become difficult controlling my chair now that my hand is weaker, plus I grow uncomfortable and need someone to shift my weight. But there's no one.

When ML comes out of surgery, I ask if she could move my hand in a particular way. She's groggy from anesthesia, can't help me, gives me a dirty look. "I can't!" she says. It sounds general and all-inclusive, like she can't take any more.

I wait. I bear up. Gradually she recovers, and we go on. But I'll never forget. I'm not proud of myself, of my inability to cope on my own, of my weakness under duress. But am I supposed to be able to cope on my own? After all, part of the independent-living philosophy is being honest and realistic about one's needs and limitations—and accommodating them accordingly. That is, having the maturity to take care of oneself. I vow to learn a lesson from this.

In the end I join an infertility support group. ML declines to go with me. I'm a believer in talk therapy; she isn't, at least not for herself. (For other people, she'll say, it's fine. A matter of personal preference.) But it is that infertility group that refers us to a reproductive endocrinologist who changes our game plan.

In May of her thirty-sixth year, I receive a phone call at home. Which immediately leads me to call the small private elementary school where she's been teaching for the past few years. I tell the receptionist it's important. When ML gets on the phone, I tell her what I've just heard. With her elementary-schoolteacher's all-in-from-recess operatic voice, I hear her yell "I'm pregNANT!"

As the months pass, I have no choice but to hire additional attendants. Dad is completely amenable and generous when I request extra *dough* (his clubby, tongue-in-cheek slang, not mine). Sometimes Dad seems more concerned about ML's well-being than mine, but probably every husband of a pregnant woman has felt something similar.

Our daughter (we had the ultrasound) is due Christmas Eve. She's late. A few days after Christmas, with no sign of contractions, we see a specialist at the hospital. (ML drives us herself.) "The baby has the cord around her neck three times," declares the specialist, wielding the ultrasound wand.

A heavy silence fills the small examination room. Again, in the movie in my mind, I'm the one who breaks the standoff. "Should we be worried?" I ask.

"Yes," he says, and orders an immediate C-section.

During the prep, with a little help from ML as she tries to lie still, I use her new cell phone—bought just for this purpose—to call Jorge, then Roger, a man I'd hired off a list from the independent-living center to stay with me overnight when necessary.

The delivery-room nurse struggles to put a gown over me. It gets caught on my chair controller, and I almost run her over before I can make her understand. After, I tell her to put my chair on manual and just push me.

She pushes me right up to where ML is splayed out and partially anesthetized. At my trusting, helpless wife's request, I begin a gentle play-by-play of what I see going on.

A few minutes later—as the delivery-room radio plays The Monkees' *I'm A Believer* ("Then I saw her face . . .")—Paula is born (named after my mother). And everything is fine.

***

I stay with ML and Paula at the hospital as much as possible. Remembering the egg-retrieval ordeal, I'm diligent about having Jorge or Roger check in with me every hour and a half to two hours. I've learned I need that, need someone to adjust my position, take me to the bathroom, or get me a sip of water at regular intervals. So I can cope over the long haul. And it works! I do not freak out this time. Self-knowledge gives me a kind of power. I wasn't sure we could do this, ML or I. But we do, and I'm proud of us both.

CHAPTER TEN

NESTING

1996-1999

"My wife made me what I am today—completely self-reliant emotionally!"

—Anonymous

"So basically she's like a single mother?" says a particularly frank (read *tactless*) friend of mine.

I had thought that myself for a time, so my answer is all worked out: "Not at all. There's more to parenting than changing diapers, you know."

Still, it *is* a crummy question. Accusation, it seems. I know my buddy is needling, but he's probably not the only one in the world likely to draw such a conclusion.

The facts are these: I don't have fantasies of teaching my kid to throw a baseball or catch a football or go fishing. None of that jock stuff. But I would like to ride with Paula on the merry-go-round, carry her high on my shoulders, build sand castles together. Stuff Dad did with me and I remember fondly. But I've resolved myself to the reality that I can't be the kind of father I had; if I try to do activities other dads do I'll fail and feel miserable, defeated. Yet just because I can't do those physical fatherly tasks doesn't mean I can't contribute.

A while back I'd attended one of those community forums at the independent-living center. A woman explained that just because you don't do things in the way other parents do doesn't make you unfit to be an actively involved parent. You just have to find your own methods, your own "reasonable accommodations." She was a wheelchair-riding foster mother who had proved her maternal chops over and over.

I don't explain all this to my alleged friend. I simply say that I have my ways of managing. In truth, from the moment Paula was born I launched a new chapter in creativity. Thanks to a startup group in Berkeley called Through the Looking Glass—which is dedicated to parenting with disabilities—I know I'm not alone in this. Learning how other disabled parents cope—what they've invented—sparks ingenuity.

For instance, I suggest ML strap a Baby Bjorn to the push handles of my chair, so Paula can ride against my chest looking either backward or forward (without killing my shoulders or upper back). We take many family walks around the neighborhood this way, with me usually whispering (okay, trying to sing) softly to Paula's curly-topped, half-asleep head.

When she's a little bigger, we hook a couple of PVC pipes between her stroller and the front of my wheelchair so I can push her in the park.

When Paula's a toddler, a photo in the Through the Looking Glass newsletter gives us our best idea yet. It shows a mother who installed a child's seat between the footrests of her wheelchair. We devise our own, simpler version. ML takes an old belt out of the closet and stretches it across the backs of my footrests, behind my calves. Paula instinctively knows what to do: She waddles toward my feet—invariably untying my shoelaces, just for a laugh—stands herself by pushing down on my foot pedals, climbs up, spins around, and sits herself on the belt, between my legs, with the back of her head basically level with the upholstery of my seat.

This becomes a favorite spot for many years, until she's big enough to ride on my lap.

My chief skill as a parent is making up silly songs and games, and telling stories, while monitoring Paula as she bathes in the kitchen sink or, later, in the tub. Or waiting at the doctor's office or on long car rides. After a while I notice something about my stories. They tend to be of a particular variety—The Bunny Who Could Not Hop or The Friendly Gorilla (Who Refused to Fight). They're all about characters who have a deficit in the eyes of their peer group. And by the end of the story we learn not to reject or discount those who seem different. Later, I graduate to Scooby Doo and superhero stories. These usually have a moral, too. Something about gumption and persistence.

No, I can't change diapers. (Wasn't really looking forward to that aspect of parenting anyway.) But I've learned how it's done, in case I ever need or want to instruct my attendant or anyone else to do it. Plus I pride myself on being a partner in the decision-making and other details. Somebody has to pay the bills and update family members on how we're doing! Those sorts of jobs fall to me. I've also devised an easy remote switch for a camera and video camcorder, to document every new tooth and other developments.

I don't kid myself. Obviously, ML has taken on a tremendous responsibility—baby and I both depend on her, and at times she bristles under the pressure. More about that later.

The pressure eases somewhat when Paula's older and I can find ways to play with her and give ML some much needed rest. We've had our sizable terrace enclosed with Plexiglas, to be baby safe, and put a small slide and climbing structure on it. It's almost like a giant playpen, the enclosed area. I go out there with Paula, keep her company, keep an eye on her, play her games, and hours can pass while ML gets a break. In time she'll go so far as to get a mani-pedi, but not yet. For now she has to remain within earshot in case something happens beyond my control.

***

Another way in which ML is not like a single mother is financially. She doesn't have to worry about making a living. She becomes financially dependent on me.

That's a curious perk of my disability. When Paula is three months old, ML's supposed to go back to work. The prospect breaks her heart. "I can't see spending all day with other people's kids while someone else plays with mine," she says.

We hatch a plan. If we let go my personal-care assistants (the new tongue-twistery term for attendants, frequently shortened to PCAs), ML can quit work. We'll end up the same economically. The money Dad sends for the hired help would go to her—or, really, stay with us—instead. She'd be taking on a lot of necessary work, and I'd be giving up a lot of independence, but it'd just be a temporary arrangement. Till Paula's in preschool or kindergarten, let's say.

***

Historically—even well into the middle of the twentieth century—certain people with disabilities were forcibly sterilized. Usually those with mental retardation. People like me were probably not expected to have children anyway.

The fact is, my disability *is* hereditary. No one else in my past had it, as far as we know, but spinal muscular atrophy is an autosomal recessive disorder; both my parents must have been unwitting carriers. Long before Paula was born, ML and I'd discussed what we'd do if our baby had a disability. Spinal muscular atrophy or any other.

"It'd be great!" I'd said. "What better parents for a crip kid than us?"

"Don't you think you're being a little selfish? You'd want to exploit our child for political purposes!"

All I'd known was my mother always said the day she'd found out about my disability was the saddest in her life. And I hated that she felt that way. I tried to understand that she'd meant she was sad because she worried about how hard my life would be. But through talks with Barbara and other leaders of the disability movement, I'd come to despise the concept of disabled fetuses being aborted simply because of their disabilities.

"If it's a painful condition, that's different," I'd allow, trying to see things my wife's way. "Then perhaps it'd be unfair to prolong its life, its suffering. But the thing is, you never know what might happen. You never know what a child is capable of."

During her pregnancy, ML had the amniocentesis to determine if Paula would be born with Down syndrome. Not that she'd necessarily want to abort; we'd agreed it was better to know in advance, to be prepared. There were no prenatal tests for spinal muscular atrophy.

Yet within months of Paula's birth, researchers in France identify SMA's genetic markers. A test (though not a prenatal test) becomes readily available. We have no cause for concern (if that's the right word; I'd've been proud regardless); Paula shows no indications of floppy baby syndrome—but ML and I go in for the test. We know I'm a carrier; if ML is, too, then our children have a fifty-fifty shot of having SMA.

Michelle, the geneticist at UCLA, seems almost excited to try out this new genetic test. She's eager to explain how it works, how she has to take a little blood from me to determine which specific strain of SMA-causing chromosome abnormality to look for, then some from ML to see if she has it. Michelle recommends testing my brothers and their wives as well.

Though the results are predictable—ML isn't a carrier, so our kids won't have SMA (but will be carriers); both my brothers are carriers, but Alec's wife is not, so no SMA for their kids either (as of this writing, Jeff isn't married)—one consequence of this genetic testing causes chills.

It's Dad. Confronted with the irrefutable proof that he's a carrier—which, of course, we'd always known—Dad is unaccountably surprised. "I always thought it was those diet pills your mother took that caused you to be handicapped," he says.

Dad is not a big one for science. Had he really held onto this cockamamie belief? Had he really blamed (or credited) Mom all along?

"Mom took diet pills?" I ask. "She told me she didn't take even an aspirin when she was pregnant. Natural childbirth, breast-feeding, all that stuff."

"It was different in those days. Doctors' instructions were different from now, and you didn't question. But yes, I remember the diet pills she took."

There's remember and there's remember. I ask him what the pills were called, but he has no recollection.

I think this is funny enough to tell ML later. Her reaction: "No wonder they got divorced." Whether she means because of Dad's resentment, because of Dad's poor memory, or because of his scientific stupidity, I'm not certain.

***

After Paula's born, Dad changes toward me. In phone conversations, he starts treating me with more acceptance and respect than before. He seems . . . less displeased. Perhaps it's because he's paying less attention to my employment status—or lack thereof—and more to baby news. Or he simply likes being a grandfather (though he already was one; Alec's wife had the first grandchild).

Whatever the reason, my becoming a father softens him.

One day, Dad tells me he's been given the name of a magazine editor who is looking for freelance writers. It's a California-based Wall Street magazine called *Buy Side*. "Not for me," he says. "I'm busy enough. But maybe for you."

This isn't grasping at straws. It's a real contact, a real name, phone number, and address. I think it's the first time Dad's actually led me to possible work, instead of just complaining I don't have any. Now that I'm thirty-four!

ML takes down the information for me (since I can't jot it down myself, and don't have a recording device handy), including the funny name *Buy Side*, whatever that means. Before I forget—without bothering to look for a copy of the magazine, which I wouldn't have found anyway because it's closed circulation—I send off a letter and résumé. That much I have down to a science; I've sent out hundreds, if not thousands, since college.

After a few weeks, hearing no response, I follow up by phone. The editor—let's call her Roberta—answers right away. She has a kind but harried voice, and she's not sure she remembers my letter. She promises to get back to me.

"If I don't hear from you in . . . what, two weeks? . . . may I call you again?" I say, having been burned before.

I don't actually count the weeks. We have a new baby in the house. Time passes strangely. When I think a goodly amount has passed, I phone again. And this time she gives me an assignment!

What she wants me to do is write a profile of the equity-research operations at an LA-based investment banking boutique. Confident I'll figure out what that means later, I ask the sort of questions I've grown accustomed to asking: Are there previous articles that would serve as good models of the style she's looking for? What would she like to see done the same or differently?

Roberta sends me a few copies of past issues. Each one contains a couple of investment-bank research-department profiles. From these examples I can almost put together a template of what she wants. I'm a good imitator, a practiced chameleon who can adapt my writing style to fit the needs of my employers. Er, I mean *my clients*.

With self-confidence akin to foolhardiness, I jump in and call the investment bank's press office, which sends me a thick envelope of background material I don't understand. When I tell Dad what's come of his lead—and thank him again for it—he says, "Send me what they sent you. Maybe I can get you up to speed."

This is the new respect I'm referring to. A level of trust. Not sure *I* trust it yet, though. I know Dad. He's going to try to take over. Typical of him not to see me as separate from him, to fail to distinguish between us.

A few days later, Dad spends about an hour on the phone with me giving me a tutorial on investment banks. He helps me draft questions for my interview, outline what to look for, what to include. It calms me down, gives me confidence. I was wrong. He's genuinely helpful. We've never had a conversation like this, one where he's respecting my intelligence and competence by sharing his knowledge, his expertise. He's at last paving a path, not burying me in the dust and mud of harsh judgments and impatience.

It's a small investment bank—hence the term "boutique." I have one primary contact to interview there; any others are optional. I'll have to interview this main person face-to-face. That scares me shitless. So far neither he nor my editor know I'm disabled.

I devise a plan of attack: I'll ask him a few questions by phone first, to establish my competence and open the relationship (using my usual speakerphone and tape recorder). Then I'll complete the interview in person, at which time—having already invested in the process—he'll dare not balk at the sight of me.

My target, Stephen, is pleasant to talk to. Some interviewees hate the press and think you're out to screw them. Others are pleased at the publicity. Stephen is in the latter camp. I imagine a fat honcho—his ecru-shirted belly hanging over his navy-pinstripe-suit pants—with a big, fake smile and a bogus-warm handshake. I'm terrified of meeting in his office.

In preparation, I don a suit (or should I say *the* suit, since I have only one) and tie. I bring a small tape recorder so I don't have to take notes, which I couldn't do anyway. I print a list of questions and clip it to a clipboard to keep it steady and readable on my lap. I try to memorize the questions just in case. Finally, I tell Jorge to stay in the reception area in case I need him. (It's better to keep him—in his soccer shorts and rock 'n' roll T-shirt—separate.)

It's a lovely, modern office in Century City. Polished light-wood walls and chrome fixtures. To be professional, I must be absolutely clear about my needs, whatever tools and modifications I require, I remind myself. Disability rights isn't about making people feel sorry for you or take care of you; if we don't want others speaking for us, we must take responsibility for knowing what reasonable accommodations we require. Or to put it another way, Mom was right: You have to speak up and ask for what you need. No one's going to read your mind.

Stephen steps out to greet me. He's a tall, lean man in his fifties, with thinning wisps of once-blond hair, khaki chinos and a blue shirt, sleeves rolled-up, with a loosened striped tie. Not at all what I'd imagined. If anything, I'm overdressed.

He offers his hand for shaking. I say, "Uh, I can't really reach out, but I'm glad to meet you." Or I intend to, but he's already withdrawn his hand. The awkward moment passes.

He leads me down the hall to a spacious office with big windows overlooking a commanding view of West LA. The office is messy, boxes stacked everywhere as if he's only recently moved in. He kindly pushes a chair out of my way so I can face him at his desk.

We exchange a few more pleasantries. He sees the tape recorder in my lap and asks if he should take it. I say okay, thanks. He places the tape recorder on his desk and pushes the record button. I'm relieved I don't have to call Jorge yet.

And then, when Stephen starts talking, something else emerges. When he gets going and gestures, his arms quiver and his hands shake. At one point the phone rings and he's positively spastic about answering it. Early-stage Parkinson's, I'm guessing.

I pretend not to notice, and he does the same of my disability. Yet as I watch him I feel a bond develop between us. Is he watching me, too?

A fellow crip!

***

For my first draft, I follow the basic structure of a similar profile that appeared in the magazine's last issue. I complete the draft a few days early so I can fax it to Dad for review. He's a kind editor, it turns out. He preserves my tone while suggesting a few small changes and asking one or two factual questions. Again, I delight in his soft but thorough touch, his not taking over. In the end, I take some of his advice and reject the rest.

Roberta is pleased with my submission and gives me another, similar assignment. This time the investment bank is in the Midwest. No budget for travel (thank God, since airplanes are difficult for me). "Just do phone interviews," she says.

No complaints, here. I don't tell her why, though I should've learned from seeing Stephen that disability is everywhere these days.

By my third *Buy Side* assignment, I'm still unsure if I've got the hang of it. My tendency is to repeat what worked before. So I send a draft to Dad.

"You don't need my help anymore" is his reply, startling me. "You know what you're doing by now, and there's nothing more I can teach you."

Such a revelatory compliment! Is he sure? Can I do this on my own? Yes, I think I can. I just didn't think it would be so easy to move Dad out of the way. Or, I realize, for me to actually let him move out of the way.

Pushing he doesn't need. He's bowing out. He's passing the baton. He's letting me "stand" on my own. In old photographs, he always seems to have a hand on me, holding me up, steadying my balance. So this is the start of a new relationship between us. Something like that moment at Stanford when I was seventeen and we ate fresh fruit from the concession stand and smiled in unison at the luminous passing coed. This is better, though. Not only does he respect my abilities, but I have a new respect for his—his skill at mentoring without taking over, a quality I didn't recognize in him before. Plus now we share an affinity for financial writing—something he doesn't have with Alec, though I always felt Alec and Dad had more in common with each other than either one had with me.

***

I never do another face-to-face interview. Not ever. Phone and, later, e-mail are sufficient. In the modern, rush-rush world, no one seems to think this odd. Most of the busy Wall Streeters I deal with are grateful to spurt sound bites by cell phone while waiting for a plane, riding on a train, or driving (soon, though, everything will have to be vetted through corporate legal departments). The days of the off-the-cuff or overheard comment at the corner bar are over, thankfully for me.

Over the next few years I become exceedingly busy churning out one or two stories a month for a succession of editors. (The magazine's name, *Buy Side*, refers to professional buyers of stocks, bonds, and other securities—portfolio and mutual-fund managers, primarily—as opposed to those who sell them, or sell information about them.) I gain a reputation as a fast, accurate, deadline-observing writer. All from a corner of my living room.

In that increasingly well-equipped corner, I work out a way for my computer to record my speakerphone interviews, which makes playback and transcription easier. No buttons to push, just icons to click. That plus the voice-recognition software contributes to my alacrity in turning around stories, which I submit by fax or e-mail. And as I gain confidence in my skills, I feel current, high-tech, telecommute-y—rather than "handicapped" by the arrangement. In fact, I'm pretty sure my disability is never detected. The magazine's offices are in woodsy northern California, some four-hundred miles away from arid, smog-choked Los Angeles, so I never meet my editors in person.

Are the famous words of Alexandre Dumas—*"rien ne réussit comme le succès,"* or "nothing succeeds like success"—true? Now that I'm an "experienced" financial journalist, Dad tries to find me more leads on work! He almost has an arrangement sewn up with one editor, but then for some reason—perhaps because travel was involved?—he mentions I'm in a wheelchair. She becomes more than upset, Dad tells me later; she's angry. "You should've informed me at the outset!" she snaps.

Nonplussed, Dad assumes she's concerned about the public face of her fledgling publication, about having someone like me represent it. I assume she's concerned about a potential lawsuit, in this post-ADA era. In any case, I'm dumped before I've started, without explanation. And Dad, incredulous, comes to experience firsthand the sort of hurdles I've been facing.

In time, another editor he knows is interested in my *Buy Side* experience and soon assigns me to write short profiles of winning stock analysts. I presume Dad's careful not to mention my defining physical feature this time.

And so I become a busy contributor to both *Buy Side* and *Institutional Investor*. They're similar magazines, with an overlapping audience, but *II* is older and more prestigious. Using its name when I call or e-mail for an interview always yields a quick response.

What's more, as the Internet bubble pushes the stock market ever higher, and demand for Wall Street news surges, I'm able to parlay my growing portfolio of published clips into opportunities at personal-finance magazines such as *Individual Investor*, *Online Investor*, and *On Investing*—all of which would evaporate a few years later, when the bubble bursts (*Buy Side*, too, eventually).

But in these dizzying Clinton years, I think how just a short time ago, when I'd lost partial use of my hands, everything I did was for the disability-rights movement. I was completely immersed in cripdom. My sense of identity is upended now as I don a yuppie guise—and become a handicap hider.

***

In 1996, when Senator Bob Dole runs against President Clinton, it's a historic moment for people with disabilities. No one with a visible disability has run for the high office since Franklin Roosevelt—and unlike Roosevelt, Dole is forthcoming about his impairment (an arm injured in wartime). It sets a political conundrum for some in the movement: Dole may be one of us, and may have been an early supporter of the ADA, but aren't Democrats better for disenfranchised minorities?

That same year, a woman with Down syndrome becomes the first person with that diagnosis to receive a heart and lung transplant. She'd been turned down at first, but hospital administrators cave to activists.

These and other milestones occur out of my tightening loop. Work and home life have become my all. "I'm nesting," I say when asked.

Once a month, I still attend board of directors meetings at the independent-living center. But my involvement is only fragmentary; doubt about its priorities and relevance are filling in the spaces. One gripe: too much emphasis on fundraising these days, due no doubt to government cutbacks.

One Saturday afternoon we're called in for a special meeting to discuss a development campaign. The executive director—an effective leader and devotee of the movement, who is nonetheless a bore—challenges each of us to name five people we can contact for donations. I get a sour taste in my mouth, but come up with my list. I even write my own dunning letter, conjuring up what the place should be, could be, used to be, and maybe would be again with adequate funds. My heart's only partly in it.

Why give to the ILC? Because it has such thought-provoking forums, which have changed my life? It hasn't had one in a year or more. When the budget became tight, forums weren't considered essential. Because it maintains a registry of potential personal-care assistants? Ever since I found Roger through the registry, before Paula was born, it hasn't been kept current. Many phone numbers are out of date, and most of the candidates are women, whom I never use. Because of the disability consciousness it raises? Alas, it's become too dependent on government funds to be as politically active as it used to be.

Besides, I've grown tired of the monolithism of the activist movement—the approach some leaders have adopted of speaking for the entire disability community, no matter how many other folks with disabilities may disagree. Usually I concur with these leaders, but not always. Take assisted suicide, for example. I continue to believe its legalization would be dangerous for people like me, but I've met disabled people who would become suicidally depressed if the opposite occurred— if the theoretical option of assisted suicide were taken away. Don't they count, too? Like many movements, "official" doctrine is trying to dictate what people should think, denying what many members actually feel. Which pretty well sums up why I've never been a joiner. I fear the group will wipe out individual dissent.

I also stop writing for the disability press, though for different reasons. I turn down assignments because they pay too little compared to what I'm making as a financial journalist. I'm still not working full-time, but rarely have enough spare time to justify extra low-paying work.

Beyond all this, the local disability community is splintering. Few of my activist friends are still around. For instance, Paul Longmore has become a professor at Stanford and, later, San Francisco State. Soon, my friend Barbara will move North, too—to be with her husband.

Barbara's wedding is a big deal. Or should I say her *weddings* (plural)? A while back, Barbara and I had a long conversation about her piss-poor odds of ever finding a husband. "I'm a disabled woman in my forties," she'd argued.

"So what? Forget the statistics. The statistics are about *other* people. They're about the past. Past performance isn't an indicator of future returns." That last being a phrase I'd picked up from the investment business.

"There's a stigma," she'd insisted. "To available men, I'm damaged goods."

"I'd marry you, if I weren't already married."

"Don't go there. I'm serious."

Sure enough, a few months later she met another activist—a man who had survived childhood cancer and now walked—and sometimes sat—with difficulty. His spine was deformed, and I don't know what else.

When they decided to get married, they faced a bureaucratic obstacle. Medicaid and its concomitant In-Home Supportive Services—a California program to help pay for attendants—places a limit of $2,000 on each recipient's savings (which is why I never qualified). But if two recipients marry, their savings threshold doesn't double to $4,000; it's reduced to $3,000, or $1,500 per person.

"We can't afford to get married," Barbara complained, fairly and accurately, "because of the stupid marriage penalty."

So the wedding was postponed. Eventually—and I don't know how they did it—Barbara and her fiancé, Dan, got an exemption. So they held one wedding ceremony as a kind of political event, complete with press coverage, and another just for friends and family. Actually, there might have been two others—one in southern California and one in northern California. I'm not sure. ML and I go to the one in LA

It's an evening service and reception. Barbara dressed up her wheelchair with regal white fluffy stuff as well as wearing an elegant gown herself. Disability style, it occurs to me, is something each of us, individually, creates every day.

The invitation said adults only, so we've left Paula home with a babysitter—for the first time. A fact that makes ML grumpy. "I feel like I've left my right arm behind," ML says when asked how she's doing.

A few years later Barbara and her husband die within a month of each other. He'll go first, from a resurgence of cancer. She from a ventilator malfunction.

Ostensibly. But I think it's at least partly the exhaustion and deprivations of grief.

***

Two years post dumping Jorge and (once again) declaring independence from paid staff—two years of having no one assisting me other than my devoted but overstretched wife—you'd better believe sparks fly in the home fires. At first, to be sure, being on our own was fantastic! The freedom to be naked in daylight hours! To eat in bed in front of the TV (*Sesame Street* and its ilk, of course)! Plus no more attendant who can't drive me anywhere without rolling down the windows to make catcalls at passing women. No more hypersensitive hired helper who picks up lunch at McDonald's every day and feels insulted when the groggy clerk doesn't understand his loudspeaker order for a "feesh fill-ette."

But all good times must come to an end, yes? So now tensions are rising. On the one hand, ML, at thirty-eight, tires of constantly balancing conflicting demands. And I, on the other, currently thirty-five, miss having someone to boss around, someone to complain about and make fun of behind his back. (That's only partly a joke. Of course it's the sense of independence that I miss most of all.) ML's working awfully hard, with nary a break. But she's not all mine, like a hired person; I'm having to make do with less help—or less attentive help.

If anyone had asked, and we'd thought about it enough to answer honestly, I'd like to believe we both we're secretly thinking, or praying, *When will this temporary arrangement end? How will we transition out of it? What's our exit strategy?*

But as usual, we soldier on devoted to our dream of doing it all, or ignorant of any viable alternatives (if, indeed, there were any). I recall one morning when I needed help dialing London (both my computer dialer and the state-sponsored free operator assistance can only handle domestic numbers). Paula, at eighteen months, is joyfully and—for all we know—dangerously tearing apart the kitchen. So ML quickly dials for me and then rushes to Paula.

When I get hold of the British stock analyst, I can interview him on my own but need wee Paula to be quiet. There's no door to close off my corner of the living room or, for that matter, the kitchen. It's really one big open space.

So that becomes ML's job of the moment—shushing the toddler. But she can't take Paula outside because (1) neither one of them is dressed yet, and (2) I might need her help again when I'm off the phone.

ML tells me later that when she enters the kitchen she's shocked to discover Paula's happily munching on a stick of butter . . . right out of the fridge! "I started to scream," she relates, laughing at the serendipity, "and then I thought, well, it's keeping her quiet. And it's not exactly poison. Fat is supposed to be good for babies' myelin sheathing."

And so, we cope. Yet another time, I go for a meeting at a fancy downtown office. ML has to drive me. It's a big money-management firm, with offices worldwide, and I'm the interviewee, not the interviewer; it could lead to steady work.

When we arrive on the fifteenth floor (I don't actually remember the exact floor number, but it was high for LA), the receptionists are thrilled to see a baby in the office! But I shoo ML and little Paula away as quickly as possible. Don't want to look unprofessional.

Afterward, I'm stuck in the lobby for an hour because ML is late picking me up. This is before we both carried cell phones.

When she finally arrives, she flatly explains, "We were nursing."

It's a phrase I hear a lot. "Where? In the van?"

"Yes. We were parked just around the corner—"

"Couldn't you have, you know, paused to come get me?"

"Well, you didn't want us around. You didn't want anybody to see the shame and embarrassment of having a nursing baby along, so . . ."

The interview, by the way, gets me a freelance assignment but no steady work.

***

Soon Paula starts preschool, which is a sort of break. Most mornings ML stays with her, but sometimes she drops me off with Paula and gets some time alone. The other preschoolers don't seem to notice the daddy in a wheelchair, though I feel awkward, especially when they're doing a hands-on art project and I can't help. Teaching Paula self-reliance, I rationalize.

Not surprisingly, little Paula starts picking up germs. Every few weeks she gets a small cold, which rarely lasts more than a few days. Because ML taught elementary school for ten years—can it be so long?—she's immune to most of these bugs. I'm not. I get sick at least every two months. And when I get sick, my very life hangs in jeopardy.

The colds themselves aren't so bad. Usually they're gone after two days. But they touch off a terrible hailstorm in my lungs. By the third day I can barely breathe. There's asthmatic tightness plus a thick gumbo of phlegm clogging the passageways. Because of my SMA, I haven't the strength to cough up even a little. If people with SMA die, this is usually the reason. Their breathing fails.

The day after Christmas I'm rushed by ambulance to St. John's hospital in Santa Monica. Breathing is so rough I'm in a panic. My trusted doctor has retired, and his replacement can only see me at Cedars-Sinai, in Beverly Hills, which is too far for the ambulance. But he has an associate at St. John's.

In the emergency room I'm given a nebulizer with albuterol mist to breathe in. It helps for a while. ML is there, of course, baby in tow. But later, I'm transferred upstairs—and swiftly forgotten. My hospital bed is left in an empty room with the door closed. ML has taken Paula home and I, lying there, have no way of getting anyone's attention.

I don't know how much time passes, but eventually I'm found. My breathing is shallow and I have a fever. A nurse struggles to put an IV in me. My veins keep slipping away, unsupported by muscles as they are. Or maybe that was earlier, in the ER, before my abandonment. I'm disoriented. The next thing I remember is the BiPAP mask—this big scary gizmo two or three big scary guys are trying to force onto my face. I can't say "no" loud enough, so I fight the mask with my tongue, pushing it away while it blows on me. I'm convinced that if it blows into my mouth it'll kill me. The big scary guys back away.

But later I awake and I'm hooked to a machine. Whether it's a ventilator or something else I can't say. I don't like it, but for two or three days I lie there and accept it. Eventually I meet the doctor who's a friend of the doctor who replaced my doctor. He makes zero impression on me.

I'm in intensive care for several days. ML visits all the time. She parks Paula in front of a TV in the waiting area, and they take frequent trips to the cafeteria and the Christmas tree in the lobby. I overhear one of the ICU nurses quizzing ML. "You are his wife?"

"Yes."

"And that is your daughter?"

"Yes. Why are you asking?"

"*His* daughter, too? Or you had another—?"

Unbelievable! I hate hospitals. No, I hate the people in them. Some of the people. I hate the way I'm treated by . . . what? . . . medical lackeys. The overworked, under-educated hospital staff. Stripped of the normal accoutrements of my life, I become the most pitiful of patients, to them. No one can see me as anything else.

Slowly I improve. I'm moved up to a double room in a regular ward. My roommate is an old man who has pneumonia. One evening I ask ML to put on the small bedside radio before leaving—soft, classical music, I suggest, so as not to be offensive. An hour later or so my roommate complains. "What's that racket!"

I apologize but he can't hear me and neither does the nurse.

I've been put on so many antibiotics I'm shitting my brains out (though I've had no solid food). Late that night, I try to call a nurse for the bedpan, but they never hear me (and my roommate, now sound asleep, is no help either). When a crew making rounds finally notices me—well, doubtless what they notice is the smell—they clean me up and change the disgusting sheets I'm lying in. "We should get him a diaper," one of them tells the other.

"No," responds the other, mercifully. "He doesn't need a diaper."

It's been five days, and lying in a hospital bed isn't good for me. I can't eat unless I'm sitting upright—there's no one to feed me anyway—and I keep being left in uncomfortable positions.

"Every time I leave you you seem fine," says ML, "but when I come back they've got you in a terrible position and you look awful again. Until I fix you."

"They won't listen to me," I say. And it's true.

After a week the personality-less doctor says I can go home as soon as I've reduced my steroid intake to a manageable level. I could've left today if I hadn't already had the high dosage. "But tomorrow," he says, leaving me hanging there.

The next morning a nurse comes around with my meds. I ask her what they are. Damn, if she isn't about to inject me with another hundred milligrams of the steroid prednisone! "No," I insist. "The doctor said I need to reduce that today."

Fortunately, ML is standing bedside that moment to vouch for what I'm saying. The nurse heads off to check her instructions. While she's gone, Paula plays with a roll of surgical tape and ML teases me about having a cross on the wall over my bed. I'm thinking about how on-the-ball and assertive you have to be even (or especially) when you're dead sick.

The nurse comes back, thanks me for setting her straight, and administers the correct dosage.

Once home and fully recovered—which takes the next two weeks—I begin to search for a new doctor. Over the ensuing months, which become years, I go through several physicians, each of whom prescribes a different regimen of inhalers, nasal sprays, and allergy pills. I should mention that I'm now paying for my own HMO, which limits the selection of doctors. In any case, I keep getting frequent respiratory infections—including one bout of pneumonia, though I manage to stay out of the hospital this time.

Finally, an article about the amazing asthma solutions at the National Jewish Health Center in Denver inspires me to phone for a referral in the LA area. From my first visit with the recommended physician—an allergist, whom I'll have to pay out-of-pocket until I can swing official HMO approval, but I'm too desperate to wait—I feel I'm in good hands. He changes all my daily maintenance prescriptions, and sure enough, the cycle of bronchial agonies ceases. Maybe it's a coincidence, but I give him full credit.

I still get sick, of course. And every time I'm in danger of respiratory failure. But now it averages only once or twice a year.

***

When the illnesses taper off and ML and I are no longer in crisis mode, an emptiness moves in like the evening fog. Soon Paula will be in kindergarten, leaving ML open-ended. She'll have time, but she won't in a way, because what if Paula gets sick and has to stay home? Or what if I need her? She still doesn't want to go back to teaching. She doesn't know what she wants to do.

My work continues, though at a more relaxed pace; somehow I'd managed to keep up despite my frequent illnesses. I did a lot of work from bed and at odd hours—waking early to call Europe, staying up late to call Asia. I'm not sure I could've done it—survived my health problems or accomplished so much—without ML's indefatigable assistance. Yet at the same time, our complete lack of privacy from each other—of time apart—has become unbearably grating.

Loud, nasty arguments pile up like multicar collisions on the freeway—frightening, irritating, damaging, and blocking forward movement. I recall thinking aloud once how awful it is to be dependent on someone with whom you're fighting, and ML's retort that having to help someone who's pissing you off isn't exactly a picnic either.

Eventually I talk her into a short spell of marital counseling. "Why does nobody give me credit?" I ask in the protected enclosure of the therapist's small office. "Everybody can see what ML brings to the relationship, but my contributions are less obvious. I handle the finances, the social calendar. I'm the anchor and the planner. I'm the motor that keeps us moving upward and onward. And frankly, I put up with her shit, too. . . . No, I don't want a medal. Just recognition."

"And what do *I* get?" ML responds. "It's never enough for you. What more do you want from me? No, I'm not a saint. If I were a saint, this would be easy. I'm just a hard-working wife and mom."

We agree to do a better job of validating each other. Which, of course, only goes so far. After our second session we come home to a particularly horrific quarrel. I don't remember now what it was about. What's crystal clear in my memory is how it ended.

After the squabble, while Paula is still at preschool, we make love for the first time in months. A few weeks later ML realizes she's pregnant.

Miraculously (aren't *all* babies miracle babies?), our fighting stops. Just like that. Like magic. Sure, some of this détente could be because I again have to hire more attendants, so I'm not left feeling so helpless and needy. And there's nothing like being pregnant to give a woman a sense of purpose and direction. But at any rate, this is the chain of events that puts an end to our torturous interdependence at last.

Come 1999, when I'm thirty-six, I'm completely oblivious to the watershed Olmstead decision of the US Supreme Court, which will free many disabled poor from forced institutionalization and springboard efforts to reform Medicaid. It's all the buzz among the disability-rights set, but I'm busy. I'm still nesting.

Miranda is born in the spring.

CHAPTER ELEVEN

THE BUBBLE BURSTS

2001-2005

"Tell so much of the truth you can't afford to have anything not true because it spoils the taste."

—Hemingway's letters (1926)

One evening, in the half-light of the girls' bedroom, I'm telling a bedtime story when my thumb slips off my wheelchair controller. The girls are curled up together on the bottom bunk—Paula, age seven, will climb to the top when it's lights-out—and I'm parked beside them. Scooby and the gang are frantically trying to capture the harrowing Pillow Monster . . . who threatens to bore them all to sleep. Our heroes are already on their second plan, and as the girls have learned by now, second plans never work! Only third plans do, and for that, the "Scooby friends" typically request a suggestion from the audience.

So when I pause to address Paula directly, she naturally assumes I'm asking for the third plan. But Miranda, only four, interrupts. "*I* know," says Miranda. "Why don't they ask the purple bat thingy!" *Fingy*, she pronounces it. (So cute!)

Miranda's been obsessed with this "purple bat thingy" since watching some God-awful video. My stories are much better, but I haven't fathomed this purple bat thingy.

"Mir*and*a," shouts her big sister, "not again! What they should do is, they should capture the Pillow Monster by offering it some candy and then calling its mommy."

"Okay," I say, unable to enjoy this banter as much as I'd like because a frisson of panic has shot through me, "but Paula, I was going to ask you something else."

I ask Paula to lift my right thumb back onto my chair's T-bar joystick. She's grown used to helping me drive my chair; my hand has continued becoming weaker and weaker. I can no longer steer left or navigate backward. At times I have her sit on my lap and just take over. She's learned to be careful.

This evening, Paula crawls over her sister, stretches toward me, and places my thumb where it should be. I can't keep it there. It falls again!

I pretend nothing's wrong and finish my story as quickly as I can. I have the purple bat *fingy* lure the monster with a plate of candy to where Pillow Mommy is waiting with open arms and the all-important, hard-heart-melting reminder that he's loved. In a twist on the traditional Scooby story, the monster is so touched he takes off his own scary mask to reveal the true, comfy, loving pillow beneath. The end. Lights out. Sweet dreams. You two are the best.

I have Paula give me a push backward as she climbs up to the top bunk, and I'm able—just barely—to round the corner back to my room. Where ML is reading in bed. "My thumb," I say plaintively.

She tries to lift it just as Paula did. It falls again. The bone-chilling realization sinks in: I've lost strength in my primary digit, the one I've used to drive my chair, roll the trackball mouse on my laptop computer, etc.

***

Once again, I seek expert advice. My beloved miracle-working allergist recommends a rheumatologist, who in turn refers me to a hand surgeon. All of whom blame my thumb's desertion from the dwindling troop of useful muscles left to me on my "basic underlying neurological condition"—namely, spinal muscular atrophy. But I've never known a body part to just up and fail so abruptly. I refuse to believe it's due to SMA. The culprit must be something new. Something new and terrible, but perhaps treatable.

While an orthotics rehab therapist tries to fit me with a custom-made thumb brace (which doesn't work), I make an appointment with a neurologist who knows about SMA. Not Dr. King Engle, who isn't available for several months. Someone at UCLA, which has a rival "muscle clinic."

The UCLA neurologist—spookily named Dr. Graves—does another round of EMG shock tests and confirms that SMA is probably the cause of my current complaint. I'm now over forty, and SMA is still rearing its ugly head.

You'd think I'd be used to it by now. And that thought alone gives me comfort, actually. Just when I can't take any more . . . any more weakness, any more limitations, any more atrophy . . . I realize I can and I will. Because I always have. I always do. I have no choice.

Eventual acceptance gives a degree of relief. It is what it is, and at least I know there's nothing I can do about it now. Nothing I could've done about it ever. I *have* to accept it. Another small but crucial piece of muscle is gone. End of story. Move on.

This phenomenon falls under the gloomy category of Aging With A Disability. I'd known this day might come—once I'd discovered my muscles were still capable of atrophying—just as I know I might someday need to hook a ventilator to my wheelchair. As my late friend Barbara had said, you plan ahead for future deterioration even as you mourn each loss. Plan and mourn: The two go together.

In a sense, I'd planned for this when I got my current wheelchair a year ago. I'd looked into alternative driving controls then. I'd made a point of choosing the chair carefully—one that could work with the latest high-tech accoutrements, unlike its predecessor, which was whatever model the salesman had said was best. This time, as an enlightened cripple, I'd gone to Rancho Los Amigos.

Rancho is a big rehab facility south of LA, famous among local crips in part because of its extensive, well-staffed wheelchair clinic. Wheelchairs aren't like cars. Most have to be special ordered, and few can be test-driven. At Rancho, I was at least able to see several different varieties. I was given options. When I was a kid there weren't any choices other than upholstery color. Everest & Jennings was the only brand. Nobody uses E&J anymore, and I'm not even sure it still exists.

I'd considered mouth controls at Rancho, as I'd seen many quadriplegics use, Christopher Reeve being the best known. There are basically two types—first, sip and puff, for those with scarce facial movement but who can suck and blow on a tube; second, a joystick that's positioned near the face instead of at hand level. The sip-and-puff type allows you to set a direction and speed, whereas a joystick is "proportional," enabling subtle gradations in both speed and direction.

I'd resisted either option. I didn't want a control literally in my face. Studies had shown a greater stigma attached to disabilities that were visible from the neck up; in fact, the least disturbing disability to the general population was supposedly low-level paraplegia—in other words, those wheelchair jockeys who had muscular torsos on top of thin, nonfunctioning legs. Hence, the cognitively or psychologically disabled were unfairly considered the lowest on the totem pole.

Which is the stupid reason I'd stuck with a hand control, knowing it might not work for long. At the same time, I saw a revolutionary new mini-joystick, invented in Belgium, that utilizes magnets instead of springs and, therefore, requires an absolute minimum of muscle strength to control. The device was so small it could be installed anywhere on a wheelchair. I should've gotten it then, but it costs about $3,000.

This, I figure, is what I need now.

With Dad semi-retired, it's my stepmother who's footing my medical and attendant bills. Even though she'll retire soon, too, she has a nice pension and has saved and invested wisely. So once I explain the situation, the funds are forthcoming.

Truly, I am lucky among cripples!

When the mini-joystick comes, I foolishly insist on installing it at hand level, not mouth level. I still have just enough wiggle left in one finger to activate it, I figure. But the installation takes so long ML has to leave me at the wheelchair tech's to go pick up the girls at school.

When we finally return home, I'm able to swing into the elevator without assistance—then, backing out, I find I need a pull from behind. Better but not perfect.

What follows is a lengthy, laborious process of customization at home—so finely tuned and patience-draining that the wheelchair techs would never do it. These kinds of adjustments can only be done at home, with constant tweaking—sometimes at five-minute intervals. Tighten here, loosen there. Move it up at the right—no, that's too much . . . My body is inconsistent, unreliable.

My wife seems indefatigable, even when I lose it. And at times the resemblance between myself and a slave driver is incontrovertible. I do not give up! I will make this chair and this $3,000 control system work!

If I thought the questions about minimum doorway width and such that Harvard presented before my arrival were grueling, this is geometrically worse. Which angle is best for my baby-weak hand? Does the shirt I wear make a difference, because of the weight of the sleeve? What about the effect of weather? (My fingers always freeze up when the slightest bit cold.)

The mini-joystick is so sensitive that standard joystick tips are too heavy. It comes with its own—a choice of a pinky-sized rubber suction cup or a cork ball no bigger than a marble. I can't decide which I like better—the cork marble extends higher than the rubber concavity, but my finger rolls off its sleek surface. So ML and I get the idea of making our own cork tip. She pops open a bottle of wine and, after a healthy belt, starts whittling the cork.

Over the next several weeks, I collect corks of various shapes and sizes, testing each one on the joystick. And not just from wine bottles, either; Chimay and other imported ales come with a cork stopper, too. (Chimay, being from Belgium—like the mini-joystick itself—seems particularly fitting.) A rough surface gives better traction than a smooth one against the pillowy tip of my middle finger, I discover. A sharp edge gives leverage.

It's maddening, all this fine-tuning. Yet what gives me emotional strength through it—besides raw necessity, the need to get it right or be immobilized—is the memory of past successes. With determination, we'd managed to have kids after four years of infertility. I'd managed to tame the breathing problems that had been plaguing me. A similar sense of mission had seen me through finding work, even if not enough of it, and, well, to finding love. In fact, my very survival owed a great deal to perseverance—the notion that problems are merely puzzles waiting for a solution.

Honestly, though, survival takes more than gumption. Flexibility is definitely part of the mix. In the end, I can make the chair work if someone positions my hand exactly right. Good enough, I convince myself. You can't wait around for perfection.

My stubbornness in preferring a hand control to a mouth control will get the better of me, however. I become increasingly homebound, afraid to try to move long distances. We stop taking walks around the neighborhood. The Internet becomes my social life. I'm afraid to visit the girls' schools without assistance. I avoid most social contact outside of home. And I crash into furniture and doorways a lot.

When I do have to go out, ML assists with the chair. It's a big tank of a thing, and not easy to push, so she tries to drive it with the mini-joystick—and frequently runs into her own shins! Ouch! This goes on longer than I'd like to admit.

***

One of the doctors who'd examined my hand after the thumb-slipping incident noticed something unexpected. My bones were dangerously thin, she'd said.

I had enough on my mind already. But eventually I bring up the question of premature osteoporosis with my primary physician—an HMO gatekeeper whose sole usefulness to me is authorizing referrals to specialists. "Eat Tums," he suggests blithely, "and here's a prescription for Fosamax."

Fosamax, in case you've never taken it, is a tricky drug. You swallow the pill once a week on an empty stomach—that is, first thing in the morning—and must stay upright without eating or drinking (except water) for a half-hour afterward. In other words, you have to be out of bed and *not* have coffee. Talk about torture. But I obey. I have bigger worries on my mind. Like how I am going to keep driving my chair.

Come spring, which is roughly six months later, I suffer terrible abdominal pain and rectal bleeding. The HMO doctor—who resembles the love child of a Nilla Wafer and a marshmallow, unfortunately—declares it hemorrhoids and recommends Preparation H. I wonder if he'd've been so blasé if I were able-bodied.

This is the last time I see or talk to this particular doctor.

I call ML's physician for a recommendation of a gastroenterologist. And I stop the Fosamax because I'm sure there's a connection. The recommended gastroenterologist—a friendly, bookish African-American guy in his forties—won't confirm the connection to Fosamax but recommends a colonoscopy. Let's fast-forward to the results: I have ulcerative colitis. It's not deadly but it's also not curable. It is, however, treatable. It's also something that seems to run in the family—my big brother Alec received the same diagnosis a year or two earlier.

I'm put on a litany of medications, on top of the respiratory and allergy stuff I've already been taking. Interestingly, steroids figure into both. Ulcerative colitis and asthma are both thought to be caused by a hyperactive immune system; if the steroids can keep the lungs and colon from becoming inflamed, the logic goes, my body won't respond by "attacking" them with painful contractions and a shitload of mucus.

Each ailment, though, takes something away. One by one they age you. Beyond whatever harm the disease itself can do, there's an impact that leaves you feeling forever winded. Then again, at least it isn't cancer. I tell myself this over and over. Still, I can't help at times feeling reduced to a needy, tormented geezer—my crip destiny catching up with me, a fate I can't escape.

I'm nearly forty-three, the age Mom was when she was first diagnosed with the cancer that took her life four years later. So I feel old . . . but sort of fortunate, too.

***

My work for financial magazines dries up. Though my earnings had doubled and redoubled over the past few years, the bursting of the dot-com bubble has put everything on hold or on the chopping block. I get assignments, but only occasionally. I take on a few writing jobs for the disability press, work I'd've snubbed a short time ago because it pays only a quarter of my old rate— plus, let's be frank, it seems to lack cachet. I don't want to be a professional cripple—someone whose entire skill set revolves around a single biological attribute. I don't want to oversee diversity at some corporation or university, or be an ADA compliance officer or employee of an independent-living center. Noble professions, all, to be sure. Only not for me. Similarly, I don't want to be a disabled writer who writes exclusively about disabilities.

Instead, given the spare time I have, I draft a novel about Wall Street excesses. I want to use what I've learned. I send the manuscript to a few agents, but nothing comes of it.

My bum hands make using the computer mouse more difficult than ever. For as long as there's been Windows, I've been using a small rollerball device that Microsoft used to make. I even went on eBay once to order as many Microsoft ballpoint mouses (mice?) as I could find. But now, even the small degree of movement *it* requires is too much for me.

The Dragon voice program does have mouse commands, but they're imprecise. And you need a mouse click to start Dragon—or, more problematically, to get it restarted when it crashes. It crashes regularly, though that may be because I like to have many windows and programs open at once.

There's another, more embarrassing reason I need to find a new mouse. As I've said, I'm having more spare time. And I'm staying home a lot more than I used to. So I'm staying at my computer a lot, with little to do. I do a lot of creative writing, but there's still time left over. So when the girls are at school and ML is running errands, or when she takes them to the park—in other words, when I'm home alone—I occasionally surf porno. After a while I become somewhat addicted to it. I have so few secrets, so little privacy, I figure I'm entitled.

With ample experimentation I discover—now that my hands can no longer manipulate my dick through my clothes—I can actually masturbate hands-free.

It takes a lot of porn, concentration, and time—and just enough strength to clinch up internally and make my dick wiggle against my shorts—but it works! It's like a wet dream when you're awake . . . only better! (Take heed, adolescent quadriplegic boys everywhere: It *is* possible.) The greatest discovery since, as a kid, before my back surgery, I learned I could suck my own dick.

But when you have too many windows open on your computer at once—and some of them are linked to questionable websites—you run the risk your computer will freeze up or crash. And with no ability to click out or restart, you're stuck. Until help comes along. In my case, that's usually my wife, though sometimes I call the building's maintenance man (the remote phone switch I have now automatically dials the operator, who connects me with any local number for free).

When help comes, there you are with the embarrassing evidence of your masturbatory voyeurism frozen on the screen . . . for all to see. It's important to the enjoyment, however, to preserve the guise of privacy—so if you're like me, you make up a simple, plausible excuse like, "Damned pop-ups!"

So: Must buy a new mouse to save me from these and other embarrassments.

I search online. This is harder than it might sound, and not just because of the variety of high-tech equipment. For me, it requires intense honesty and self-reflection. I still think of myself, at times, as "the boy who can't walk" or "the boy in a wheelchair." In other words, my legs don't work. In truth, my arms never worked all that well either, and now my hands are crap. As with my job search early on, I must face facts about the extent of my impairment.

So in the end I resign myself to a mouth-controlled computer pointing device. There are several brands—basically joysticks you can move with lips and click with forced puffs of air. Only one costs less than a thousand dollars, however. It's only $800 plus shipping and handling.

A local dealer sells me his old demo model for a hundred. I take it home and try it. *Voila*! Like magic. Now I can truly operate the computer totally hands-free! Porn sites and all . . . which are suddenly much less appealing.

***

But money remains tight. I rely on credit cards more than I should. Even my monthly checks from Social Security abruptly stop coming. Worse than that, I receive an unbelievable notice to reimburse the agency for overpayment!

I'd been receiving benefits I didn't deserve, apparently, for the past several years. Social Security wants me to pay back no less than $70,000. I can only laugh. $70,000! What's really funny is, I'd been telling Social Security it was overpaying me for years.

Years earlier, not long after ML and I tied the knot, when I was embedded in the disability-rights movement, an activist pal had told me to keep my wedding a secret or face the consequences.

"Too late for that," I'd scoffed. I'd already written about being married in a few of my published pieces.

"Be prepared for a big, nasty bill, then."

As my late friend Barbara had put it, it was the marriage penalty—not unlike what caused her to postpone her own wedding. The checks I'd been receiving since college—since Mom died—were Social Security Disability Insurance Survivors Benefits; only *unmarried* survivors of deceased parents are eligible.

Once I heard this, I debated what to do. I figured I was already in hock for something like $7,000—why go to Social Security and invite trouble? So I tried saving my monthly checks in a separate account. That way, if and when Social Security got wise, I'd have a chunk of money ready to send in. But alas, I only managed to save a few hundred bucks.

Plan B (or my "second plan," as I might've put it in a story to my kids) was to tear each new check in half and send it back. This almost worked. (I should've known better; second plans never work.) Social Security responded with a letter asking for an explanation. Which I answered promptly and candidly. I said I could no longer accept benefits because I'd been earning more money—and was married.

So when a man from Social Security phoned, I expected a scolding, perhaps, or at least an official termination. Instead, in a friendly tone, he asked a series of questions. How much was I earning? How much did I spend on personal-care help and equipment to keep me employed? He didn't ask about my marital status at all.

Again I answered honestly. There was a long pause. Then he came back: "By my calculations, you don't need to return these checks. I'm going to have them all reissued to you. And your future benefits will continue. You see, we count your employment-related expenses against your earnings . . ."

"You're sure?" I interrupted.

That was as far as I pressed. Perhaps the rules had changed. I didn't want to push him too hard or volunteer extra information.

So the checks kept coming. I couldn't stop them, even while other disabled people I knew—who really could've used them—couldn't get the benefits they deserved no matter how many times they applied or how hard they argued.

Why had the inscrutable federal agency caught up with me *now?* No way of telling. Naturally, I file an appeal; I accept the termination but argue against the outrageous repayment, saying I wasn't at fault and had never sought to deceive. But my appeal is denied—partly, I'm told, because I can't honestly claim *inability* to repay. I still have savings from the sale of the New York apartment all those years ago, which generate dividends and interest I live off of. The best I can do is negotiate a repayment schedule. That activist pal who'd warned me all those years ago that this day might come said the terms could be pretty reasonable.

"How much you wanna pay back monthly?" asks the charming, molasses-voiced woman at the repayment office in Chicago or Philadelphia or somewhere.

"A hundred?" I blurt.

When she says fine, I catch myself. That was too easy.

"Actually, would fifty be enough?" I say.

It is. How low could I have gone? Then again, even at this rate I'll have to live to a hundred to be debt-free. And I don't want to saddle my heirs with too much liability. But maybe by then the marriage penalty will have been overturned.

***

I write a short essay-cum-exposé about this injustice, but I can't decide whether my tone should be ironic or irate. The piece never gets published.

I try writing about other things that perplex, obsess, or incense me. Isn't that what writers do? Observe the world and filter their experiences through their artistic sensibilities? I no longer want to be just a mouthpiece for the cause—penning angry, semi-official disability-rights essays. On the other hand, I don't want to hide my disability either. I can't deny that the movement has raised my consciousness, as we used to say; my perceptions are informed by my exposure to and affinity for the group. But now they are *my* perceptions, my take on events, not expressions of groupthink.

I'm moved in this way by the unexpected death of a friend from the independent-living center. Fred was a fellow board member—a tall, jocular, spinal-cord-injury survivor who drove an oversized electric wheelchair. Was he even thirty? He was full of bonhomie suffused with evanescent sorrow, frequently asking me how I cope. I regret that I usually just smiled and shrugged him off. (Well, I can't literally shrug, but you understand.)

When I hear he's dead, I immediately wonder if he killed himself. He was never maudlin, yet plainly unhappy with his life as a cripple. He talked a lot about the good old days—sports, girlfriends. I thought he was just going through an adjustment phase, his accident being fairly recent.

At Fred's memorial service, my skin begins to seethe. His loved ones keep talking about his pre-accident athletics . . . almost as if they miss those old days more than anything, as if perhaps they liked *him* better then, too. Someone, maybe his father, concludes with something like, "Now he's in a place where he can run and jump again." And there's a tearful murmuring of agreement from the front row.

When I come home, I rush to the computer and write about this in a kind of mental fog. How dare his family deride or, worse, negate his post-accident life? If he had suicidal ideations—fantasies of escaping this world for a better place, a place where he could again be what he once was, the young able-bodied man his family wanted him to be—it's no wonder! I save my draft under the title "Suicide"—and promptly forget about it.

It's only several months later, after I hear an invitation on NPR to submit short essays for a program about strongly held personal beliefs, that I rediscover the old file with the provocative name. *Suicide*? What's this . . .?

I revise, polish for radio, cut to the required length, and prepare to e-mail it to NPR. Why not? What've I got to lose? Before clicking send, though, I tweak the title to something more descriptive . . . something more evocative and less *provocative* . . . and come up with the rhetorical question: *Are there no wheelchairs in heaven?*

The next day an NPR editor writes back. She asks if I'm willing to do a little rewriting. She suggests I play up the idea of no wheelchairs in heaven and lose the suicide angle, since we can't actually prove anything.

I'm grateful for the feedback—the speediness of the reaction, too, which is always a good sign. I don't understand at first what she means, what she wants, but in the end I conclude she's right. Brilliant, even! A great editor!

Yes, I've tried to combine my artistic sensibilities with my disability consciousness to craft something uniquely mine, something authentic. At forty-three, I feel I finally have the maturity to be genuine. It may even be the first time I've written from the heart.

But . . . well, if I'm an artist, I'm one who's devotedly practical. If it can get out over the NPR airwaves, I'll do what she asks. This isn't really about suicide, though I still think that ties in; it's about the stabbing hurt I felt at that memorial service. Leave out the politics. Keep it personal, which may be a stronger political statement anyway.

I revise and resubmit. An interminable two weeks passes. Had my optimism been premature? Then comes the phone call . . . can I be at the studio in two hours?

The girls are in school, so ML and I pile into the van—a minivan now, thanks to my stepmother Barbara's generosity, with a lowered floor, seats removed, and a folding ramp—and rush to NPR's Culver City studio.

***

The three-minute monologue airs a few weeks later, one December morning. I'm embarrassed by the breathy tinniness (or do I mean "tininess"?) of my voice. Not very macho. Then again, why should I sound macho? I'm not a pitchman or an actor. I sound like what I am—a person with a disability. Still, I worry someone at *Institutional Investor* or *Dealmaker*—which still throw a little work my way every now and then—will find out.

By the time I get to my computer that morning I've already received e-mail about it. "I am a Leadership Coach [and] your piece inspired me and encapsulates for me what coaching is all about—optimism and perspective," goes one message. "I teach a reading assessment course," says another, "[and] have always tried to instill a sense of respect for 'disabilities' . . . I would like to have a copy of your story to share with my students on the first day of class."

For the next several days they keep coming. The editor of a poetry website wants to post a transcript of my prose. A congressional aide who uses a wheelchair writes to say, "It's wonderful to know that I am not alone." A man in Vermont says my words changed his "outlook on the day if not the year" and asks if he can "help spread your point of view." I've made a parent of a child with Down syndrome "feel better," and touched someone with a loved one who died from muscular dystrophy. I even inspire a woman who heard me online in Germany.

Requests for reprints pour in. My piece is used in disability-awareness courses, tolerance and diversity newsletters, spiritual seminars. A rabbi in New Jersey asks to use it in her Rosh Hashanah sermon—and posts my words in the temple lobby!

Perhaps the most humbling message of all, forwarded by NPR, concludes: "I'm still an atheist, but Ben is a god to me."

I get a little swoony from all this. From the effect I'm having on people. I'm used to being told I'm inspirational. Heard that one all my life, but usually for doing nothing but existing. For living life on wheels. This feels different, deeper. I've actually touched people with my words. Is this, I wonder, what's meant by finding your "voice"?

And if I can reach people this way, I'd better be damn careful about what I'm saying. For almost instantly I wonder where this will lead. Will I have access to this soapbox again?

Lost so long in the marginal marshlands of the un- and under-employed— even at my busiest, I'd always had the sense I could do more, work harder—I'm desperate to be needed professionally. Desperate for respect, for direction, for solid ground. Will NPR provide at least a stepping stone?

An answer of sorts comes not long after. My editor all but commissions a follow-up. Can you perhaps do something for Valentine's Day about you and your wife? she suggests.

Thrilled to, of course. Yet a cautious note sounds within me. I'm familiar enough with disability history to know the dangers in drawing too much attention to oneself, one's personal life—the risk of being called not just inspirational but heroic, an overcomer, an exception. I can't speak for all disabled people—and wouldn't want to, for they are a motley crew—but don't want to separate myself from the pack either. I'm just one of many, after all. It's a funny thing that tends to happen when one crip does well. People say wow, what a strong person, what an admirable individual—instead of questioning their prejudices about all the *other* people with disabilities.

It's like the old "you're a credit to your race" line. Commend the individual while insulting his tribe.

This puts me in mind of a true story Dad once told me. As a young man, he got in a conversation with an older gent on a park bench. Knowing Dad, he probably asked questions and listened to the old man rant. Dad seems to have a journalist's interviewing skills in his DNA—not a hard-hitting political journalist's, perhaps, but a human-interest reporter's. He can engage anybody in conversation, and even in his eighties he's accosted by strangers as a sympathetic ear for their political ramblings.

This particular park-bench geezer apparently veered onto an anti-Semitic tangent. "The Jews are to blame!" he told Dad. "It's all the kikes' fault!" And Dad apparently nodded, humored the guy—but did not run away. I might be remembering wrong, but I get the impression Dad came back to the park bench day after day to continue the conversation. At any rate, at some point Dad said to him, ever so calmly, "You know, *I'm* Jewish." And the man reportedly waved a hand in the air and replied, "Yeah, I suspected. But you're different."

None of us is one thing alone. We're all a hodgepodge. I can neither conceive of myself as not having a disability, nor imagine not being my parents' child. I am an ex-New Yorker, a Harvard graduate, a husband and father, a professional writer, and a person with a disability. I am all those things, but none of them is me. Not entirely.

***

After the Valentine's broadcast, I receive more e-mail. One long one in particular touches me. It's from a young woman who's engaged to a man in a wheelchair. "[You're] a beacon of hope for me and a special boy that holds my heart in his hands. [Your story] gave me so much hope for my and Kyle's future. It showed both of us that it can be done. Dreams that we have can be attained. It really was a gift to both of us."

I also get a few offers for public speaking.

So I keep pitching ideas to NPR, and though there's a lull for nearly a year—due, I presume, to management and budget issues—more broadcasts follow. (A few of the pieces that don't make it on air alight in print.) And I wonder, have I finally successfully married the two sides of my identity? The educated professional journalist and the disabled man. Or rather, should I say, the educated professional *is* the disabled man, and vice versa? Am I at last one whole person, encompassing the diverse aspects of my life?

━━━ ● ━━━

THE GHANAIAN CONNECTION

2006 AND BEYOND

"You see, really and truly, apart from the things anyone can pick up (the dressing and the proper way of speaking, and so on), the difference between a lady and a flower girl is not how she behaves, but how she's treated."
—George Bernard Shaw, *Pygmalion*

One dewy morning in the midst of this NPR hubbub, I'm trying to get my latest attendant to position my hand correctly over the mini-joystick. I become impatient with him, until I realize it's not his fault.

Since Miranda was small, we've had a new tactic on the attendant front. I've hired a young man to work two hours every morning, which is generally when I need the most help. He gets me washed and dressed and in my chair and ready for the day, seven days a week. Then ML takes over.

Since it's only a couple of hours, I don't have to try so hard to find the right person. I hire a young Filipino we'll call Stanley, who also works part-time at a sheltered workshop for retarded adults. I found him through an ad I'd placed on Craigslist.

Stanley follows my instructions—or does his best to—but this morning I cannot work the mini-joystick. It's almost literally the last straw—the last finger I could still move, could still use to power my chair, on an otherwise lifeless hand, has quit to join its useless partners. So the time has come.

I contact my wheelchair mechanic, Hamid—or try to. His company has vanished. Thanks to Google, I track him down in Burbank. Highly motivated to get this taken care of as quickly as possible—since I hate having to rely on others to push me, like when I was a kid—I explain what I want and urge him to meet me ASAP. He suggests a garage in Burbank he's using as a temporary office.

I arrive first thing the next day, as the morning fog is lifting. Hamid presents me with a piece of black plastic. "We can attach the mini-joystick to this collar," he says. "You hook it around your neck, near your mouth, and there you go."

I swallow hard. He's a tall, muscular man with a beer belly, looking rugged but friendly in old Levi's and a navy sweatshirt. I have no choice but to trust him. "Okay, let's do it."

I like this collar concept. The less hardware on my chair the better. Plus it has a vaguely futuristic feel to it, like Bluetooth cell phones, which are new then. Yet like all repairs and adjustments with wheelchairs, it's never as simple as it sounds. First Hamid has to order a new collar; his demo is cracked and unsafe, he says. And he'll need a doctor's prescription, to go through insurance—

"Screw the insurance. How much can a plastic collar cost?" I say.

"More than you'd think." He looks it up on the computer and announces it's something like $175. I'm in shock, but more than that I'm in a hurry. I say I'll pay for it out of pocket. I'll even pay extra to have it FedEx'd.

Three days later when I return, Hamid gets down to work detaching the mini-joystick from my armrest and installing it on the plastic collar. I wish the collar were more elegant—leather lined, or something—but it'll do. Hamid's garage is open to the outside air, and the weather has turned. Hot, dry Santa Ana winds have replaced the humidity, making everyone's nerves as brittle as yellow leaves.

In less than an hour Hamid's done. He straps it around my neck, saying, "You might want to put some moleskin around the edges. Some people find 'em too sharp."

Why am I not surprised? There's always something stupid about every wheelchair design. "How'm I supposed to drive this?" I ask when he has it attached. The joystick hangs about two inches below my lips.

He pulls the collar tighter, which doesn't help. Stanley looks on. He's working late today, since he usually leaves as soon as I'm in my chair. Till now he's been standing off to the side staring at the windy crystal-blue sky. Innocuous, but not exactly helpful.

"It's supposed to be up *here*," says Hamid, fiddling with the collar's front bib. "Most people press their tongue against the inside of their lips to push the joystick."

The thing still hangs too low, but I figure I'm smarter than it is. "Foam," I say.

At the back corner of the garage, thick gray Styrofoam is piled up on shelves. I've been staring at it, wondering why it's there. I ask Hamid to fetch a small piece and place it under the bib, between my chest and the collar. He gets the idea.

A moment later, I'm extending my lips a la Mick Jagger and tentatively connect with the mini-joystick's jagged cork tip. It works! My chair clicks into action.

"There you go!" says Hamid.

Stanley lopes over toward me. "Y'okay?"

The foam slips out from under the collar and I'm again immobilized. But now I have something to base hope on.

Once back home, I wait for ML. I don't have much faith in Stanley's fine-tuning abilities, plus he's overdue to go home. Besides, ML is and has always been my best mechanic. I explain my vision to her. She cuts variously shaped wedges of the thick foam Hamid's given me and sticks them to the back of the collar with mounting tape. We spend a good amount of time trying different configurations. The physical work isn't strenuous, just monotonous.

Once we've raised the mini-joystick just enough, and managed to keep it balanced and reasonably secure, I give it a test drive. Our hallway walls bear the telltale marks of a crashing wheelchair.

After a couple of days, I'm getting the hang of it. Only problem is outdoors. On uneven terrain, my head easily rolls from side to side, causing me to lose contact with the cork or press against it too hard and lose control of the wheelchair. What I need is a way to stabilize my head that's not too permanent, since I don't want my head frozen in one place all the time.

I have an idea. I order sheepskin grips from a medical supply catalog I sometimes use. They're actually made for crutches, but when they arrive I ask ML to attach them to my headrest, one on either side. (Another Velcro marvel!) The idea is to provide just enough resistance to keep my head in the right place. The solution isn't perfect. I learn to be careful on bumps and inclines, which can still upset my head and cause me to crash the chair. But under most circumstances I feel as nimble as Fred Astaire. I can go left, right, forward, and backward—and any infinitesimal degree in between—with ease.

Thus ends several years of halting, circumscribed mobility. Indeed, I become more maneuverable than ever, and so mobile I soon have to get my own cell phone.

***

It's around this time that I find Jerry, the UCLA student from Ghana who asks nonjudgmental questions about my life and gets me thinking about it from a different perspective—how I've coped and why I remain optimistic. If in my NPR commentaries I did successfully synthesize my educated professional self and my wizened-yet-vulnerable disabled self into one whole person, can I do it again? And can I do it better?

Those were short, four-hundred-word pieces. What about something longer? Can I reflect on my past in that same light, with similar honesty? Without worrying about whether my words are politically correct or push disability-rights dogma? Without worrying about whether it'll undermine my Ivy League yuppie identity or my disability-activist cred? Can I prove I really am able to be both at once—yuppie and cripple— at length, without caring about who finds out my secrets and what they think of me afterward?

The truth might not come off as cool as I'd like, just as my radio voice isn't as macho as I'd hoped. But is that going to stop me? Do I care anymore about seeming cool?

The first time I'd tried to write a book about my life, I had to hide it in fiction—embarrassing fiction, in which I'd brazenly attempted to be the disabled JD Salinger or something. The second time, a kind of thinly veiled therapy to cope with our burgeoning fertility struggle, was so far from the truth as to be completely divorced from my disability. And my third go at writing a novel, also bereft of disability, was a cynical, impersonal, and half-baked exploitation of my Wall Street knowledge. These were efforts to establish some other identity. This time I'm set on being authentic and heartfelt.

I try to sort all this out and explain my conversion—my coming to terms with writing honestly about my life—in a creative essay that's published in Newsweek's "My Turn" column under the headline, "It's just a wheelchair, not a Batmobile."

Other columns follow—in the *Chicago Tribune*, *USA Today*, and elsewhere.

And then, at last, I give myself permission to spend two hours a day writing not just short pieces but—pretentious as it sounds—a memoir. On the second day, I'm hooked. It comes easily, quickly. Two hours a day isn't enough. All this has been bottled up inside me for so long, most of my life.

I stay with it, interrupted only by the occasional magazine assignment. Or so I think.

***

Though Jerry's with me only two hours a day, the sense of security he affords me emboldens me to go a step further. Or maybe it's the voice inside me, telling me I need more autonomy—or more accurately, that ML and I must once again do the hard work of becoming less interdependent. Two hours a day of paid assistance isn't enough.

On their next visit, I ask Dad and Barbara for a temporary hike in financial support. I'd like to offer Jerry more hours—he's nearing graduation, so it's a definite possibility—to give ML the freedom to figure out what she wants to do with her life *separate* from looking after me. If she returns to teaching, she'll have to update her credentials first. That's a process. And teaching would be a major commitment, she points out; she'd like to remain available to the girls and to me.

I want to say she doesn't need to worry about that, but I have to admit she's being realistic.

"Sure," says Dad. "How much is enough? Take all the time you both need."

"Really?" I'd misjudged him. Did I remember to say thank you?

I hire Jerry full-time. ML works on her résumé and makes inquiries. She decides to look for something part-time and close to home. There's a large independent bookstore down the street (gone now, like so many others), and one afternoon she walks in with her résumé. It's not hiring, but next door is a luxury gift boutique where a friend once worked. By the end of the week she's hired there, about ten hours a week, which suits her fine. It's her first paying job in ten years. She knows nothing about retail but finds she likes it. What's not to like? She's working with a small group of kind, smart women in a clean, aromatic setting among beautiful home decor, objets d'art, and stationery. Soon her hours are increased and she gets a small raise.

***

Just as her job and my memoir are beginning to take shape, I have a terrible run of diarrhea (so to speak). Day after day it goes on. I take Imodium round-the-clock to try to avoid accidents. I've been eating yogurt and bananas, taking the probiotic powder my gastroenterologist recommended, and a pharmacopoeia of colitis drugs—all apparently to no avail. "It's a flare-up," says the doctor. He puts me on a high dose of prednisone.

With the prednisone, I immediately feel better. The abdominal cramping eases and my mood improves tremendously. This, I know, is a common side effect of prednisone. It causes a kind of euphoria. But the diarrhea doesn't stop. Weeks pass. I don't know how much weight I lose, but I can see my jawline for the first time in decades. This is not a good kind of skinny. Looking back at the pictures from the time, I appear older, my skin paler, my hair thinner than now—even several years later.

Since my original diagnosis of ulcerative colitis, I've had a few of these flare-ups. Usually a few weeks of prednisone takes care of them. ML says prednisone makes me snappish; I say it makes me impatient. It also makes me hungry, which is good because I'm losing so much weight. Except my body isn't processing the food properly. It just goes through me. My regular doctor—the internist I switched to after switching out of the HMO—says I've become anemic, among other ailments. Of course, that could be because of losing so much rectal blood (mixed with the diarrhea).

If you think chronic diarrhea is bad, try having it in a wheelchair. I'm not able to rush to the toilet. To sit on the john, I have to be lifted into bed, stripped, and then lifted onto the rolling commode. So suffice it to say this is a messy, disgusting period of my life. I'll spare you further details.

In December 2007, shortly after I turn forty-five, Dad and Barbara are visiting for a long pre-holidays weekend. Friday, they take the girls out to dinner and give us money to go out somewhere ourselves. ML and I haven't gone on a date in ages, but we're both too tired to go anywhere and decide instead on delivery from a favorite neighborhood restaurant. I have the filet mignon—I remember it clearly because it's the last meal I'll eat for the next seven months.

That night, I spend painful hours on the toilet. Early the next morning I call my gastroenterologist, though it's Saturday. He's on-call. He wants me to check into Cedars-Sinai immediately. Dad agrees to take me so ML doesn't have to. Kissing Paula and Miranda (ages eleven and eight, respectively) goodbye, I say I'll be home by Wednesday. That's what the gastroenterologist told me. I may have betrayed their trust forever.

At the emergency room, which is where the gastroenterologist told me to go, Dad and I talk about books I haven't read and movies I haven't seen. Neither of us can believe we're in the ER because I seem so hale and hearty. And indeed, I feel fine. The daytime excretions have stopped. It's just every night the diarrhea returns.

Dad likes the idea of my writing a memoir. He can hear the excitement in my voice when I talk about it. He tells me he's learned an "astounding figure"—more than two-hundred-and-fifty-thousand books are published in this country annually. Surely, he says, there's room for mine. And I flash back thirty years, when he was perhaps more frustrated with life, with his own career. He took me to the big Barnes & Noble store in the Village for the first time. "Look how many books there are!" he'd growled. "Who in hell needs another one?" Trust Dad to buck the trend and become more optimistic in old age!

In time I'm shown to a hospital bed. I still feel pretty good. But a day later, after the exploratory surgery that will lead to the removal of my colon, my doctor will explain that the prednisone masked symptoms—fever, for instance—of an advanced C-diff infection. That's *Clostridium difficile*, to those in the know—a severe bacterial infection of the colon. There's no telling how long I'd had it—and the longer you wait to treat it, the worse it gets. Mine had gotten very bad. (Diarrhea meds like Imodium might've made it worse, too.)

The only antibiotic certain to treat it now is Flagyl, a type of metronidazole to which I'm allergic. I know I'm allergic because my first gastroenterologist prescribed it, along with the original diagnosis of ulcerative colitis. My tongue swelled like a balloon.

For me, the worst part of the surgery is the intubation. Intubation makes me unable to speak. Since I can't signal with gestures, it renders me utterly powerless. Warned this is going to happen, I have the surgeon phone ML immediately. It's the middle of the night. Nevertheless, she understands my concern and hops out of bed, leaving the girls home alone, and rushes across town to the hospital. She can't dissuade the surgeon from intubating me, however. He insists it's necessary for my survival.

I come out of surgery with a colostomy bag and no way to talk. ML, the only one who can read my lips, keeps vigil beside me in the ICU round the clock. Several days pass. She tells me she's stashed the kids at her brother's and taken a leave of absence from work. She brings my usual prescription meds and nebulizer machine, in case I get into breathing trouble. Which is likely if I spend too much time lying down, especially after surgical anesthesia, which tends to deposit phlegm in the lungs. She is quite plainly my lifeline.

After two or three days the tube is removed from my throat so I can talk, and I gradually emerge from the medically induced fog. Hospitals are rough on me. Even as I'm restored to solid food, I can't eat well in bed. My atrophied muscles feel weaker than ever. And now that I have this literal sack of shit affixed to my belly, I can't put on my usual abdominal brace, which supports my breathing—my diaphragm—when I sit upright.

In a medical catalog, ML finds a similar abdominal brace with a cutout for a colostomy bag. Meanwhile, she suggests cutting a hole in my old brace. But the doctor doesn't give me permission to get out of bed. I was only supposed to be here a few days and it's a week already. It's practically Christmas and I'm thinking about my kids.

I tell the surgeon—during the two minutes he tarries at my bedside before seven AM—that I have two small children I'd like to be with over the holidays. Cedars is a Jewish hospital and maybe he doesn't understand. He says I've developed a fever.

On the eighth or ninth day I finally talk him into letting me go, provided I fill a prescription for Zithromax, to handle whatever is causing the fever. It's Christmas Eve. So desperate am I to leave that I urge ML to throw me in my chair and drive home as fast as possible, though I'm having trouble breathing. It's only because of poor abdominal support (I hope). Whatever the cause, I know I'll feel better in my own bed. She does what I ask. And sure enough, though I'm desperate for air by the time we get there, I do breathe better in my home bed. My whole body unwinds internally, and I feel victorious! Free of the hospital gulag! Home for Christmas!

Our sister-in-law brings the girls home and, before leaving, congratulates us on our "Christmas miracle." For dinner, we buck holiday tradition and order mild Indian food to be delivered. I manage to eat a few bites of naan. Then I want to sleep.

In the middle of the night my gut starts aching. Gas, I figure, a common consequence of eating lying down. I wake ML and ask to roll onto my stomach. It's my best position for sleeping, plus it should help with the gas.

"You can't go on your stomach anymore," she reminds me. "You have a colostomy there."

"But . . . I have to. Come on, you can do it."

How foolish I was. I should've listened to her. Five minutes after turning over, my stomach is hurting worse than ever. I need to roll back. For an interminable duration I try rolling this way and that way . . . It's four AM when poor sleep-deprived ML (she'd spent the past few nights in a hospital chair) notices my colostomy bag is filling with blood.

In a panic, she drains the blood into a jug—and it refills again. She calls 911.

And so, within hours of my return home, an ambulance rushes me to the UCLA emergency room, which is closer than Cedars. I remember telling the ER doctor, "My wife will kill me," since I'd made her take me home and roll me, against her better judgment. I remember ML's showing up, having told the kids to get up and open their presents without us. I remember the persistent pain in my gut, and being wheeled in a bed to a small room with a TV I can't see. I remember lots of people hovering around me, and I vaguely remember wanting to roll over again. ML says I asked for my mother, which I now know is typical of hospital patients facing imminent death.

The next thing I can conjure from memory, I'm accidentally onstage during a performance of *Wicked*. My mind is copying a surreal scene from a sitcom I'd watched weeks earlier. Everybody is gawking at this idiot who's fallen onto the stage. I can't get off stage. I can't get out from under the bright lights. Then a curtain closes—or opens. Regular light seeps in. And Dad is there, gazing down at me. Behind him, ML. My stepmother Barbara and both my brothers—Alec and Jeff—too. It's like the final scene in *The Wizard of Oz*—my whole family surrounding my bed. But in this case it's a hospital bed.

They're asking me if I recall passing out, if I know I've been in the hospital for several days. But again I can't talk. Tubes in my throat are gagging me. I try to get a focus on my surroundings, but I don't have my glasses. A maze of hallways with TV sets mounted high, that's my impression. Alec asks if I want to watch *Law & Order*. I try to make a "no" face.

I also remember thinking about an article I'd recently written for one of the disability magazines about computerized communications equipment for people with multiple disabilities—screens that give you a choice of words to generate sentences which the computer will speak. This is what I need now, I figure. Communications equipment. I try desperately to relay this.

Dad and Alec recite the alphabet, waiting for me to blink to indicate a particular letter, to spell out what I want to say. I'm too woozy and can't spell. My mind keeps wandering.

Here's what I learn later: I had internal bleeding, which led to septic shock. I nearly died, at forty-five years old. If ML hadn't been there to insist I was "full code"—the opposite of "do not resuscitate"—the doctors might've given up on me.

The internal bleeding was from the colon surgery I'd had the week before. The surgeon at Cedars had left a tear somewhere inside me, which became infected! Hearing I might not make it, ML had called my family. Dad, Barbara, and Jeff were on vacation in Mexico and flew back to LA immediately. Alec came from New York. The girls were back at my brother-in-law's.

But this is far from the end of it. I remain in the ICU for the next three months—only vaguely aware of the markers of time, passing events such as the Super Bowl, Valentine's Day, the Oscars, the presidential primaries, even ML's birthday, all of which vanish into a black hole in my consciousness-memory— most of that time unable to talk. Dad, now eighty, stays with me nearly every day and ML every night. She's given notice to her employer, who kindly sends a gift basket and promises to save her job; she's also secured a live-in babysitter for the girls.

Where would I be without my loving family? What happens to those who have no one, who are alone? I shudder to think. And though I'm not a praying man, to this day I try to thank God every night.

To explain why I'm stuck in the hospital for so long is almost impossible for me. It's too grueling, too recent, too vaporous in my mind. I know I develop multiple pneumonias and scattered blood clots, pass in and out of consciousness. There are many wonderful, attentive, and patient healers, who matter more than they're ever told—if you're one of them, reading this, I'm forever in your debt—and sadly, an equal number of unpleasant or downright scary ones. The attending physicians imply I might never fully recover, might not ever get my old life back, might end up permanently in an institution—perhaps the kind the disability movement is fighting to "free our people" from.

But in March I do return home, three months after being whisked off in the night by ambulance. Though not back to my old life, not at first. For the next six months I spend most of my time in a rented hospital bed at home, with a series of clueless nurses. I use a rented ventilator off and on till mid-May, when my ability to breathe becomes dependable. I have a tracheostomy in my throat—a version of which remains to this day—and require phlegm to be suctioned. Through July I have a feeding tube inserted into my nose, through which cans of milky, unflavored pabulum must pass, my only source of nourishment. At one point I weigh less than ninety pounds, a good thirty or forty pounds off my usual weight in pre-diarrhea days. And I sleep at least twelve hours a day, through August.

My recovery is only partly a matter of regaining strength. It's also got to do with weaning off meds (which is something no one tells you!). I'd been put on so much stuff in the hospital—digestive facilitators, blood-pressure regulators, and so on—that even the doctors lost track. They just kept refilling them. Gradually I acquire the presence of mind to ask my primary attending physician directly, "Do I still need Norvasc? May I stop taking Protonix? Do I still have to monitor my oxygen levels and pulse rate twenty-four/seven?"

In this way, one by one, the trappings of my hospitalization are shed. And with fewer drugs in my system, I become more alert, more awake, more in charge.

***

There is one other vestige of my hospitalization I'd be remiss to omit: an open pressure-wound near my ass, where my tailbone protrudes. It takes another year—and several specialists to examine and treat it—before it closes up sufficiently. ML still tends to the scar.

During my convalescence, as at the hospital, no one else looks after me like my wife. All the fine details that keep me from slipping off the precipice: Am I getting the right meds on the right schedule? Is the feeding tube kept clean and unblocked? She gets so good at it that the home nurses ask if she's a doctor! And ML does all this despite sleeping only intermittently on a leaking inflatable mattress squeezed into a corner of our bedroom.

Come August, I know I have to make a break. I know I won't ease back into anything resembling my old life; I'll have to seize it, reclaim it—colostomy pouch and all. It'll be different from before, to be sure—since I now have a permanent colostomy pouch and small tracheostomy—but I'll figure it out. With ML beside me, I know I can do it.

***

When we at last say goodbye to the desultory nurses, it feels like a big step. I start looking for an attendant again—someone more skilled than I've needed in the past, but still not a nurse. A man hired by me to follow my directions, unlike the home nurses who work for an agency and almost uniformly treat me as if I were incapable of managing my own care.

To hire an extra-competent attendant will require extra money. Barbara, my stepmother—retired now, but apparently in good financial shape after a long and loyal corporate career—offers however much I need. I'm speechless at her generosity, especially thinking back on what seems like my lifetime of ingratitude.

When I was in the hospital, Barbara helped ML with the bills. Not just paying them (the total exceeded a million dollars—most of which Blue Shield absorbed) but coping with the flood of paperwork. ML was overwhelmed—unable at first to access my online bill-paying accounts, then struggling to figure out which I had on automatic payment and which I didn't. In the course of this, Barbara discovered how much credit-card debt we'd been accruing. And not, I hasten to add, from fancy dinners, extravagant shopping sprees, or vacations. Just basic expenses. (My half brother, Jeff, deserves grateful applause too, for handling my e-mail correspondences in my absence.)

Barbara's generosity engenders an unexpected side-benefit: Knowing I'm well taken care of, Dad stops worrying to death about my finances.

***

During my illness, on good days, I thought a lot about the memoir. I couldn't write, but wanted to. Conjuring up my real-life identity provided an anodyne escape from the latex-smelling tubes and incessantly whirring, beeping machines. I drafted chapters in my head, hoping to memorize them. I was eager to return to the task that had enraptured me.

Afterward, resuming the writing proves not so easy. Back in my chair, back at my computer, I first tend to my magazine work. I'd had to cancel a few assignments when I dropped out unexpectedly, and I'm eager to reestablish myself, get back in the game. There's nothing quite like nearly dying—to harken again to that Churchill quotation about missing an assassin's bullet—to make you feel reborn.

On the other hand, my second life is haunted by the specter of vulnerability. It's as close and constant as a shadow. What will happen the next time a dangerous illness befalls me? Will I have the strength to get through it? Come November 2008, I turn forty-six. Who knows how many good years I have left? I'm filled with a hunger for life but also an indelible sense of caution. A mild form of posttraumatic stress disorder, perhaps?

In any case, the need to write about my life takes on a new urgency.

***

Knowing how good it feels to be free from the clutches of hospitalization—and I seriously doubt I would've recovered so successfully anywhere but at home, under my wife's tutelage—I feel a special affinity for the current thrust of the disability movement: deinstitutionalization. In 2005 President Bush initiated a program—which President Obama expands—called Money Follows the Person, which basically mandates that any state funds for care of disabled people in institutions shouldn't be jeopardized if and when the person transitions to at-home, community-based care.

Not that the old struggles for equality, accessibility, and integration are ended. They aren't. But now they've moved into the courts, to a large degree. Lawsuits go on all the time. Veterans of the movement—who taught me so much—sometimes seem to forget how far we've come. We no longer have to agitate for a seat at the table. We're there, or at least in the door—we're part of the debate now, a political contingency.

When my daughters' school recently announced plans for a Diversity Day, for example, I immediately e-mailed the organizer to make sure disability was included in the mix of racial, religious, gender, sexual-orientation, and other issues under discussion. I was prepared for a fight—but found that two other folks had already volunteered to lead disability-awareness sessions!

At the same time, many younger folks with disabilities tend to take the cause for granted, failing to realize that those accommodations we see every day—wheelchair lifts on buses, ramped curbs, etc.—didn't magically appear out of the kindness of people's hearts. They came only after hundreds, possibly thousands, of patriots protested, got arrested, and sued for fairness.

Medical and technological advances clearly deserve a big chunk of the credit for my survival to date. But the disability movement shook me into figuring out my place in society. It showed me I'm part of a larger group—and a history—of people with all manner of deformities and impairments, and educated me on my civil rights. It rescued my self-esteem by introducing me to Disability Pride. Whatever I accomplish will not be despite my disability but *with* it.

Indeed, I couldn't tease out my disability-related experiences from the rest if I tried. I haven't had any other kind.

***

A few months after I've hired a new attendant and started getting my life back together, Dad comes around for a visit. At eighty-one, he's mellowed but still sharp. He remains in remarkably good health, despite a lifetime of loathing exercise and loving desserts. He travels, attends the theater, reads a lot, sees every movie, volunteers at a local community center, and does some creative writing.

In many ways, I realize, he's living more like I do.

I still can't believe how he uprooted—moved into a hotel for months!—to look after me in the hospital. I can see now, as a parent myself, that it's not so much that he or my mother ever held my disability against me or viewed it as a mark of shame or failure; they merely wanted to do whatever they could to give me the best possible opportunities.

Unshackled from financial obligations, thanks to Barbara, our relationship is finally free to evolve beyond all that. Dad sits back on my sofa and we talk. He likes to converse. I ask him about the past. He tells me about his childhood, his relationship with his parents, what it was like when he met my mother, and—most startlingly—how sometimes he thinks back on their marriage fondly.

He's become philosophical, and a better listener (with hearing aides, that is). Dad talks to me like an old friend, no longer a problem he must solve. And I no longer feel threatened.

"It's risible," he grumbles one afternoon, with a chuckle, still impressing me with his vocabulary, "when people tell me, 'Eighty-one? That's not old!'"

"As if 'old' were a dirty word," I say.

"It's the patent absurdity of it! Eighty-one *is* old."

It's become a regular part of his curmudgeonly idiom, scoffing at the silly pleasantries people utter absentmindedly. But this time, to me, he's struck a profound chord. How many times have I heard niceties such as, "We're all disabled in some way" or "I don't even think of you as disabled"? They're intended to convey kindness and acceptance, I guess, or to cheer me up. To my ear, though, they always sound squeamish, as if the concept of *disability* were so distasteful you have to sugarcoat it.

I ask Dad if this is what he means and he denies it. Still, I can't shake the sense that he feels patronized, even insulted, by such remarks. Haven't I heard him lament that he shouldn't have to "think young," as strangers keep commanding? He says he's entitled to move slowly, to spend long afternoons in a rocking chair or need a seat on a crowded bus or even doze off in the theater—without feeling guilty about it. "Sloth," he's joked, "is no longer a sin at my age. It is a well-earned privilege."

Dad is just being witty, I'm sure. Yet, in his old age, he and I have a lot more in common than either of us has ever realized before.

"Do you ever run out of stamina?" he asks me. "It's hard for you to work all day, isn't it?"

"Not when I'm writing," I answer truthfully. "Running around, meeting people—that tires me."

Though neither of us says it, I believe we share the idea that my writing from home instead of working in a busy office might've been the right job for me after all.

***

There's one more loose end. ML has been on leave from work since her abrupt departure nine months ago when I was hospitalized. She, too, uprooted to be by my side! And now we're both a little nervous about what comes next. Am I really stable enough for her to return to work (if she even has a job to return to)?

I have to wean myself off ML's custodial care just as I did the ventilator and all those meds—and I suppose she must wean herself off of caring for me so intently.

With my new attendant, I reassure her that I'll be okay and she should go back to work. Reluctantly, she approaches her old boss. The boss is welcoming, but the business has changed. The shop is now half what it was. It's become a high-end stationery store and nothing more. Not ML's favorite part of the business.

But next door, in a space the old store used to occupy, a new gift boutique is opening. And there ML finds some of the same kind and stimulating people, the same aromatic candles and winsome decor, she knew from before. She's hired on the spot—just a few days a week at first, but that soon grows to as many hours as she wishes.

In summer, Alec and his wife and their two daughters visit from New Jersey. We meet at Universal Studios (their idea). It's been two years since I last saw his family—and I haven't seen *him* since the hospital—but after remarking on how the kids have grown, etc., we fall into place, into our traditional roles.

In the slow-moving ticket line, I confront Alec about something that's on my mind. "Buzzy, we might be here all day. If I need to go to the men's room, you'll be able to help me, right? I realize it's something you've never done. Mom and Dad always tried to protect you from feeling responsible for me—"

He squints as if trying to comprehend, but maybe it's just the sun in his eyes. "I've never done that," he says. "You . . . you want me to hold your dick? You'll have to tell me how."

Buzzy is still Buzzy. But he's not stupid. He understands my request, that it's logical and reasonable. I don't take him up on it, however. I monitor my liquid intake throughout that day, though it's blazing hot. Still, maybe next time. If I can articulate my unique perspective, my specific access needs and frustrations, he might be receptive in a way he couldn't be as a boy.

These days, I have one full-time attendant during the week and three part-timers to cover evenings and weekend mornings. But any day, any one of them could show up late or not at all. ML still fills in a lot—I suspect neither of us would be comfortable doing otherwise, at this point—and works a five-hour shift five days a week at the shop. (I wonder how her version of these events would differ from mine. She declined my offer to preview the manuscript.)

Our girls—both teenagers now—amaze me daily with their intelligence, talent, and beauty (and height!) . . . though you never stop worrying.

The progress of our lives can be derailed at any moment—by another medical emergency or, for that matter, any number of other disasters. They are merely interruptions, I believe. So far, I've always been able to bounce back.

And indeed, ML and I are both growing older, more fragile. Yet whatever happens, I know we're a good team. Deep in my osteoporotic bones and atrophied muscles I feel we were designed for each other. We keep planning, mourning what's lost, celebrating what's gained, and then going on. That's just the way our lives are.

Try not to be too jealous.

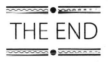

THE END

Acknowledgments

Thanks go to Skyhorse's Tony Lyons—my old pal—and Yvette Grant for their invariable and undeserved kindness, clarity, flexibility, and understanding.

To my indefatigable agent Lauren Galit, this simple appreciation doesn't do justice. Lauren, you are unmatched in loyalty, steadfastness, and plain-speaking honesty. I don't know why you stood by me all these years, but I'm glad you did!

Others in the biz were also crucial in their individual, encouraging ways. Among them: Jennifer Lyons, Bonnie Nadell, Diane Mancher, and Lynn Goldberg.

I owe a great debt to Lillian Trilling for keeping me sane by helping me tease out the various insanities that were clogging my brain. Honorable mention goes to Danny Rothenberg for "getting it." And of course—beyond family and friends (Facebook friends, too!) who've stayed in my corner sometimes against all reason—I must thank countless others both within and outside the disability-rights movement, others too numerous to mention.

The influences on this work are also myriad. Let's just say if I hadn't read Frank McCourt and Mary Karr and Augusten Burroughs and on and on, I'd've been surely lost.